ORTHOPAEDIC POCKET PROCEDURES

NOTICE

ORTHOPAEDIC POCKET PROCEDURES

General Orthopaedics

Courtland G. Lewis, MD

Clinical Professor of Orthopaedic Surgery
University of Connecticut School of Medicine
Farmington, Connecticut

McGRAW-HILL
Medical Publishing Division
New York Chicago San Francisco
Lisbon London Madrid Mexico City Milan
New Delhi San Juan Seoul Singapore
Sydney Toronto

The McGraw·Hill Companies

GENERAL ORTHOPAEDICS

1 2 3 4 5 6 7 8 9 0 DOC/DOC 0 9 8 7 6 5 4 3 2

ISBN 0-07-136985-6

This book was set in Times Roman by V&M Graphics, Inc.
The editors were Darlene Cooke and Nicky Panton.
The production supervisor was Catherine Saggese.
The interior text designer was Marsha Cohen/Parallelogram.
The cover designer was John Vairo.
The index was prepared by Jerry Ralya.
R.R. Donnelley was the printer and binder.

This book is printed on acid-free paper.

Library of Congress Cataloging-in-Publication Data

Lewis, Courtland G.
General orthopaedics / Courtland G. Lewis.
p. cm.
Includes bibliographical references and index.
ISBN 0-07-136985-6
1. Orthopedics. I. Title.

RD731 .L43 2002
616.7--dc21 2002190249

INTERNATIONAL EDITION ISBN: 0-07-121257-4

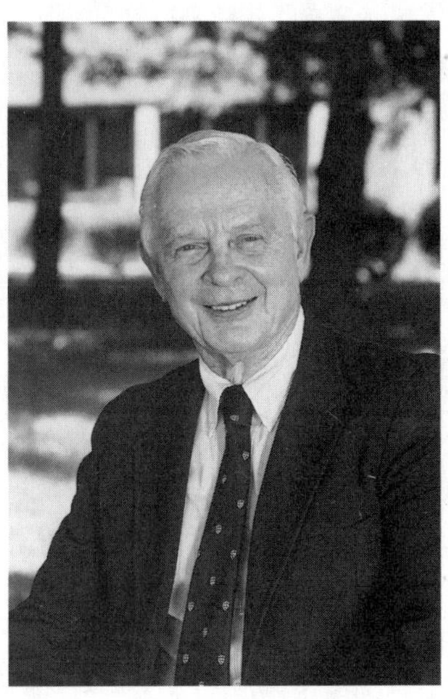

We dedicate this manual to the memory of

DR. HARRY R. GOSSLING,

Co-founder & Director of the University of Connecticut Orthopaedic Program,
Professor of Orthopaedic Surgery,
Department Chair,
and role model.

BE A DOCTOR FIRST. . . . Dr. Gossling epitomized the classic physician—dedicated to the welfare of his patient, committed to lifelong learning, and patriarch of his orthopaedic family. He taught us to heal.

CONTENTS

CONTENTS

IN ALPHABETICAL ORDER

PREFACE

In celebration of the 25th year of the University of Connecticut Orthopaedic Program and the graduation of its 100th resident, the alumni and faculty offer a guide we hope you will find helpful. Whether you are reading this on paper or in PDA format, our goal is to create a portable resource for you. Some background on anatomy and approaches, alternative treatments to consider, and guidelines for perioperative care—with room to jot down notes on the vagaries of different surgeons. The procedures are drawn from the operative logs of UConn residents over the last several years to ensure they are relevant. They are coded according to the *American Medical Association's* CPT system, which orthopaedic residents will use throughout their careers to report and bill for procedures. They are cross-referenced against ICD-10 diagnostic codes, which relate the underlying condition to a given procedure.

Whether you are an orthopaedic resident, physical therapist, or other health care professional, we hope that reviewing any given topic will generate more questions than it answers, encouraging you to read and inquire in more depth.

At UConn, we pride ourselves on how we care for patients. We hope you will find our advice by clinicians for clinicians helpful.

COURTLAND G. LEWIS, MD
Farmington, Connecticut
October 2002

ACKNOWLEDGMENTS

My thanks to Carolyn Bedula, department administrator at Hartford Hospital and orthopaedic "mother" to many residents over the years, for her invaluable assistance in organizing this manual. Our thanks also to Darlene Cooke, Susan Noujaim, and Nicky Panton at McGraw-Hill for their professionalism, patience, and persistence in bringing this project to fruition.

CONTRIBUTORS

Thanks to the following alumni and faculty of the University of Connecticut Orthopaedic Program who have contributed to this manual:

MICHAEL ARON, M.D.
Hartford, Connecticut

MICHAEL ARONOW, M.D.
Farmington, Connecticut

ERIC BENSON, M.D.
Bedford, New Hampshire

BRUCE D. BROWNER, M.D.
Farmington, Connecticut

ANDREW CAPUTO, M.D.
Hartford, Connecticut

SAMUEL D'AGATA, M.D.
Hanover, Pennsylvania

JOHN FULKERSON, M.D.
Farmington, Connecticut

GREGORY GALLANT, M.D.
Doylestown, Pennsylvania

JOHN GRADY-BENSON, M.D.
Hartford, Connecticut

ROBERT GREEN, M.D.
Hartford, Connecticut

W. JAY KROMPINGER, M.D.
Hartford, Connecticut

WILLIAM MANNING, M.D.
Hyannis, Massachusetts

MICHAEL MIRANDA, M.D.
Hartford, Connecticut

THOMAS MURRAY, M.D.
Portland, Maine

MARY LYNN NEWPORT, M.D.
Farmington, Connecticut

CARL NISSEN, M.D.
Farmington, Connecticut

CHRISTOPHER OLCH, M.D.
Bremerton, Washington

GREGORY POMEROY, M.D.
South Portland, Maine

ROBERT QUINN, M.D.
Hartford, Connecticut

VINCENT SANTORO, M.D.
Hartford, Connecticut

BRIAN SMITH, M.D.
Hartford, Connecticut

R.J. SULLIVAN, M.D.
Hartford, Connecticut

JERFFREY THOMSON, M.D.
Hartford, Connecticut

H. KIRK WATSON, M.D.
Hartford, Connecticut

RICHARD ZELL, M.D.
Chappaqua, New York

P A R T I

GENERAL

DRAINAGE OF HEMATOMA OR SEROMA

CPT code **10140 incision and drainage of hematoma, seroma, or fluid collection**

ICD-9 code **998.1 hemorrhage, hematoma, or seroma complicating a procedure**

INDICATIONS

Painful collection of fluid causing pain, fever, compromise of skin, circulation, or neurovascular function.

ALTERNATIVE TREATMENTS

- needle aspiration
- sclerosis of seroma with tetracycline or other agent

SURGICAL ANATOMY

- typically, a seroma develops after 1 or 2 weeks as the body forms a serosal lining
- once there is a lining, aspiration alone often does not prevent reaccumulation

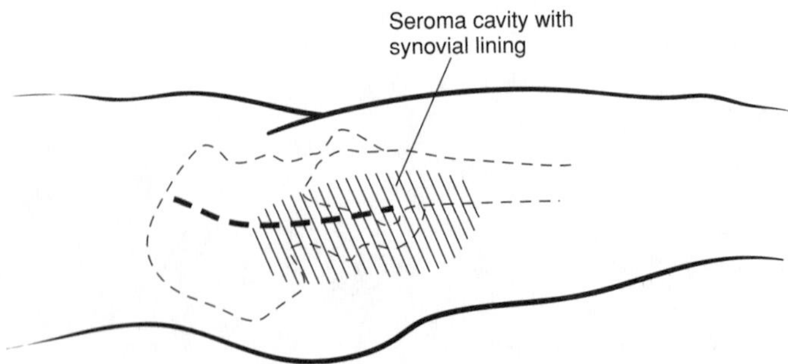

APPROACHES

Surgical Techniques

- incision through previous surgical approach or in Langer's lines
- must excise the entire serosal lining to prevent reaccumulation
- close over drain and leave drain in place until there is minimal (<25 mL per shift) drainage; vacuum drain is preferable
- maintain compressive dressing for at least 2 weeks to prevent reaccumulation

REHABILITATION

- for lower extremity, may bear weight to tolerance
- avoid active or passive range of motion of adjacent joints until dressing is removed
- isometric exercise is permissible during the healing phase

NOTES

INCISION & DRAINAGE OF WOUND INFECTION

CPT code **10180 incision and drainage; complex, postoperative wound infection**

ICD-9 codes **730.00–730.09 osteomyelitis, periostitis, acute osteomyelitis**
996.66 complications with infection or inflammation due to prosthetic device
996.67 complications due to screw, rod, or bone stimulator

INDICATIONS

Abscess or known wound infection requiring incision and drainage. Surgical debridement of infected wounds is a principle learned many times over throughout the history of warfare and in civilian settings.

ALTERNATIVE TREATMENT

Antibiotic suppression

SURGICAL ANATOMY

- depends on location

APPROACHES

Surgical Techniques

- principle is the complete removal of all infected and nonviable tissues
- with a sinus tract, instillation of methylene blue the day before surgery may be helpful (viable tissues resorb dye over 24 hours and nonvital tissues remain stained)
- if incision present, use for debridement; if a sinus tract is present, it must be excised *in toto*
- for bony involvement, the principle is debridement to bleeding bone; therefore, a tourniquet should not be used for this part of the procedure
- use of high-speed burring requires cooling with water to prevent necrosis of bone and nidus for bacterial recontamination
- in general, osteomyelitic wounds should be left open for healing by secondary intent; closure *per primum* can sometimes occur but is a violation of basic surgical principles; ask "why?"

POSTOPERATIVE MANAGEMENT

- use of perioperative antibiotics is bacteria and host dependent; it should be viewed as a decontamination procedure after true surgical debridement
- be aware of potential medication cross-reactions, particularly between sulfonamides and warfarin therapy

- duration of treatment with intravenous and oral antibiotics is highly variable; there are no prospective studies indicating appropriate duration of therapy for osteomyelitis

REHABILITATION

- treatment depends on site; if significant bone is resected at the time of debridement, consideration of possible stress riser formation is important
- infected soft tissues respond best to immobilization; therefore, unless restoring function is critical, short-term immobilization (1–2 weeks) should be considered

COMPLICATIONS

- recrudescent infection
- non-union

NOTES

DEBRIDEMENT OF OPEN FRACTURES

CPT code **11012 debridement skin, subcutaneous tissue, fascia, muscle, and bone**

ICD-9 codes **805.10–839.9 open fractures**

INDICATIONS

Open fractures or open joint injuries

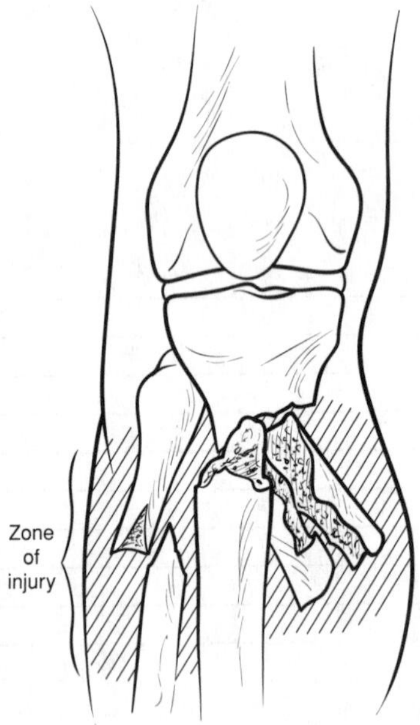

SURGICAL ANATOMY

Variable: avoid damage to nerves, vessels, tendons, and ligaments during exposure and debridement.

APPROACHES

Use extensile approaches to gain maximum access to wounds extending to deep structures. Random location of traumatic skin wounds may require adjustments in approach. Longitudinal incisions to extend wounds allow adequate exploration and debridement.

Surgical Techniques

1. limited excision of skin edges (3–5 mm) and longitudinal extension of traumatic wounds to permit adequate exploration
2. liberal removal of contused, crushed, or debris-contaminated fat
3. open fascia as necessary to decompress compartments
4. remove devitalized muscle (nonbleeding, noncontractile, discolored, or friable)
5. use instruments to remove any foreign material including small specks of dirt imbedded in soft tissue
6. remove devitalized bone fragments without soft tissue attachments; remove devitalized portions of bone that do not bleed and/or are heavily contaminated
7. copiously irrigate the wound with saline; avoid high pressure direct lavage which may drive debris into tissue

POSTOPERATIVE MANAGEMENT

1. limb elevation (at level of heart)
2. pain management
3. repeat operative debridement for severe wounds (24°–48°; schedule at initial debridement)
4. serial dressing changes
5. limited duration prophylactic intravenous antibiotics (24°–72°)

REHABILITATION

- early joint motion and muscle activity
- prevent contractures (especially equinus)

COMPLICATIONS

- bleeding
- nerve and vessel injury
- compartment syndrome
- soft tissue infection
- osteomyelitis
- sepsis

SELECTED REFERENCES

Behrens FF. Fractures with small tissue injuries. In: Browner BD, Jupiter JB, Levine AM, Trafton PG, eds. Skeletal trauma, vol 15. 2nd ed. Philadelphia: Saunders, 1998:391–418.

Blick SS, Brunback RJ, Poka A, et al. Compartment syndrome in open tibial fractures. J Bone Joint Surg 1986;68A:1348–1353.

Gustilo RB, Anderson JT. Prevention of infection in the treatment of one thousand and twenty-five open fractures of long bones. J Bone Joint Surg 1976;58A:453.

Tscherne H, Gotzen L. Fractures with soft tissue injuries. Berlin: Springer-Verlag, 1984.

GENERAL

SUBUNGUAL HEMATOMA

CPT code **11740 evacuation of subungual hematoma**

ICD-9 codes **923.3 fingernail or thumb**
924.3 toenail

INDICATIONS

Severe pain

ALTERNATIVE TREATMENTS

- "benign neglect" and usual nail loss

Incision

- directly over the hematoma

APPROACHES

Surgical Techniques

- position: directly over the hematoma

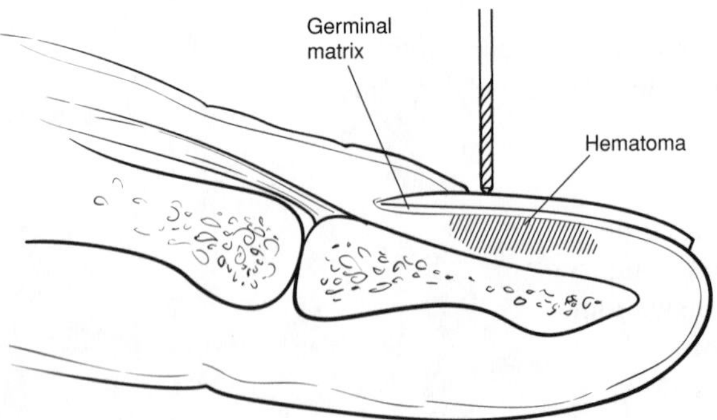

- methods:
  - scalpel or drill
  - heated paper clip
  - battery-operated bovie cautery
  - sufficient opening to permit adequate drainage
  - avoid germinal matrix

POSTOPERATIVE MANAGEMENT

- apply ice
- volar splint

REHABILITATION

- return to activity as tolerated

COMPLICATIONS

- insufficient opening for adequate drainage
- infection
- beware of underlying phalangeal fracture with the creation of a technically open fracture

NOTES

EXCISION OF INGROWN NAIL

CPT code	**11750**	**excision of nail and nail matrix, partial or complete (e.g., ingrown or deformed nail), for permanent removal**
ICD-9 codes	**681.11**	**onychia and paronychia of the toe**
	703.0	**ingrowing nail**
	703.8	**other specified diseases of the nail**
	755.7	**specified anomalies of nails**

INDICATIONS

Symptomatic ingrown toenail. Complete excision is reserved for multiple recurrences.

ALTERNATIVE TREATMENT

Soaks, accommodative shoe wear, or cotton wisp under the ingrown nail

SURGICAL ANATOMY

- nail plate: toenail itself; consists of layers of keratinized cells
- nail fold: skin overlying proximal, medial, and lateral nail plate
- lunula: white semicircular area at the proximal aspect of the visible nail plate, just distal to the nail fold
- germinal matrix: produces the nail plate; located mainly under nail folds and lunula
- sterile matrix (nail bed): responsible for nail plate adherence, not growth; located under the distal central nail plate

Incision

- partial excision: none or longitudinal into proximal nail fold
- complete excision: medial and lateral longitudinal in nail folds

APPROACHES

Surgical Technique

- digital block
- separate the nail plate from the nail matrix and nail fold

- partial excision: remove medial or lateral 10% of the nail plate
- ablate underlying germinal matrix (curette or phenol)

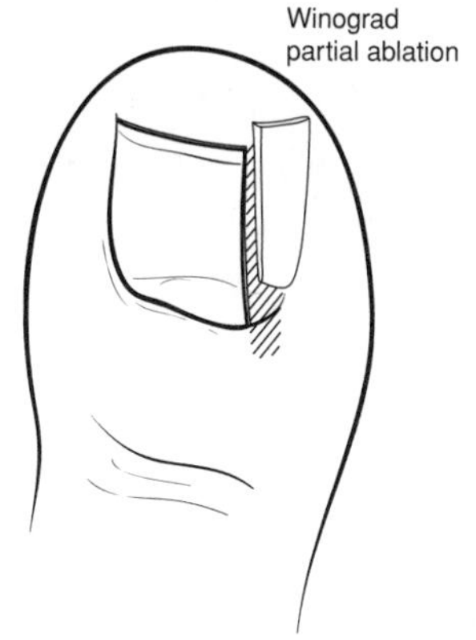

- complete excision: remove the nail plate

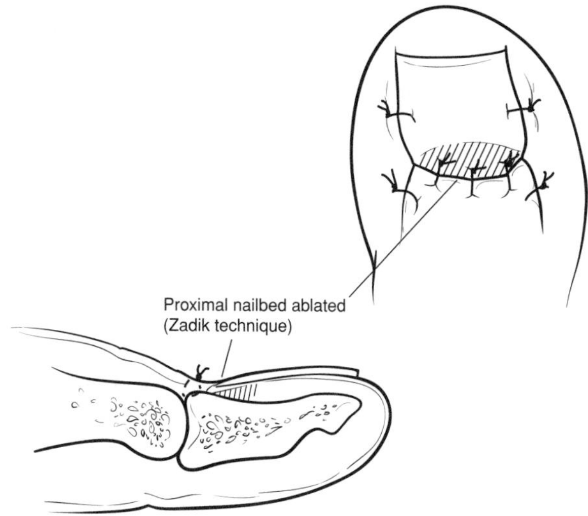

- remove germinal matrix (including the deep layer of the nail folds)
- sew skin to the sterile matrix

POSTOPERATIVE MANAGEMENT

Compressive dressing for 24–72 hours

REHABILITATION

- weight-bear as tolerated (WBAT) in surgical shoe
- partial excision: twice-daily saline or epsom salt soaks for 2–3 weeks

COMPLICATIONS

- recurrence, which increases with partial excision
- infection

SELECTED REFERENCES

Winograd AM. A modification in the technique for ingrown nail. JAMA 1929;92:229–230.

Zadik FR. Obliteration of the nail bed of the great toe without shortening of the terminal phalynx. J Bone Joint Surg (Br) 1950;32:66–67.

NOTES

GENERAL

LOCAL SOFT TISSUE FLAP FOR OPEN FRACTURE

CPT code **14020 adjacent tissue transfer or rearrangement, scalp, arms and/or legs; defect ≤ 10 cm²**

ICD-9 codes **874.10–897.10 open wounds**

INDICATIONS

- open wounds
- contracture release

ALTERNATIVE TREATMENTS

- free flaps
- muscle-pedicle flaps

SURGICAL ANATOMY

- location dependent

APPROACHES

- random pattern flaps

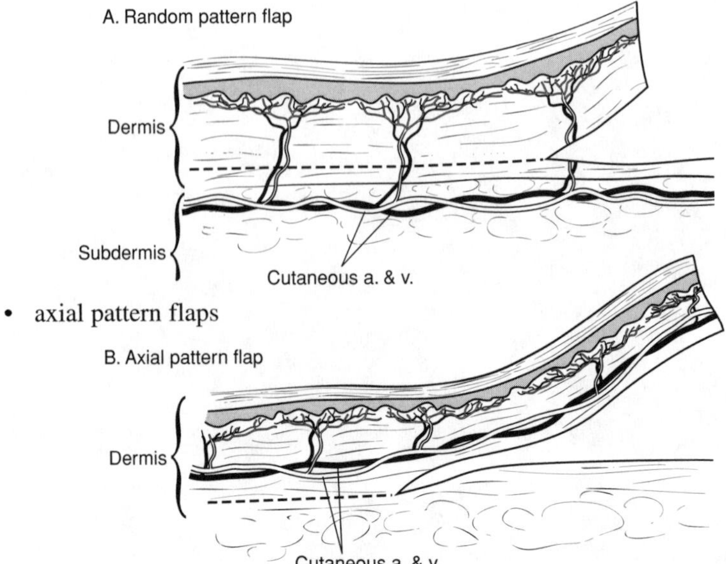

- axial pattern flaps

- free tissue coverage for "remote" lesion

C. Free tissue transfer

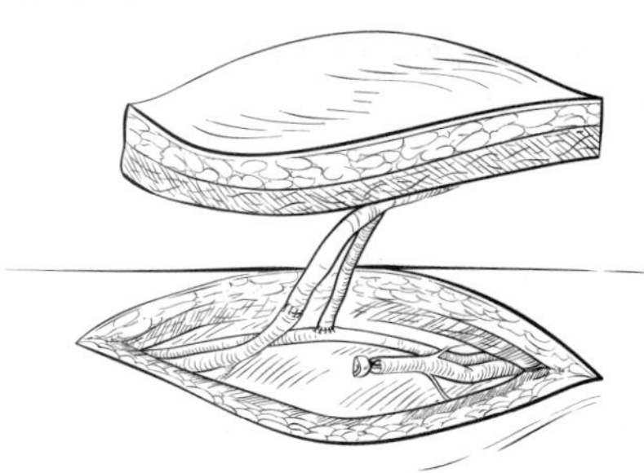

Surgical Techniques

- transposition flap
- rotation flap
- advancement flap
- Z-plasty

POSTOPERATIVE MANAGEMENT

- nonocclusive, nonpressure dressings (permit drainage)
- splinting of joints crossed by repairs
- limb elevation (at or above heart for venous outflow)
- limited duration antibiotic prophylaxis
- splint to avoid contractures (especially equinus)
- suture removal in 7–10 days

REHABILITATION

- early mobilization of unaffected joints and early muscle activity
- increasing periods of dependency to restore vascular tone

COMPLICATIONS

- complete or partial flap necrosis
- infection

SELECTED REFERENCES

Sherman R, Ecker J. Fractures with small tissue injuries. In: Browner BD, Jupiter JB, Levine AM, Trafton PG, eds. Skeletal trauma, vol 16. 2nd ed. Philadelphia: Saunders, 1998:419–448.

Yaremchuk MJ, Brumback RJ, Manson PN, et al. Acute and definitive management of traumatic osteocutaneous defects of the lower extremity. Plast Reconstr Surg 1987;80:1–12.

FULL-THICKNESS PINCH GRAFT

CPT code **15050 pinch graft, single or multiple, to cover a small ulcer, tip of a digit, or other small open area**

ICD-9 code **879.8 wound, open skin**

INDICATIONS

- small, open skin wound
- originally described by Jacques Louis Reverdin in 1869 and rarely used

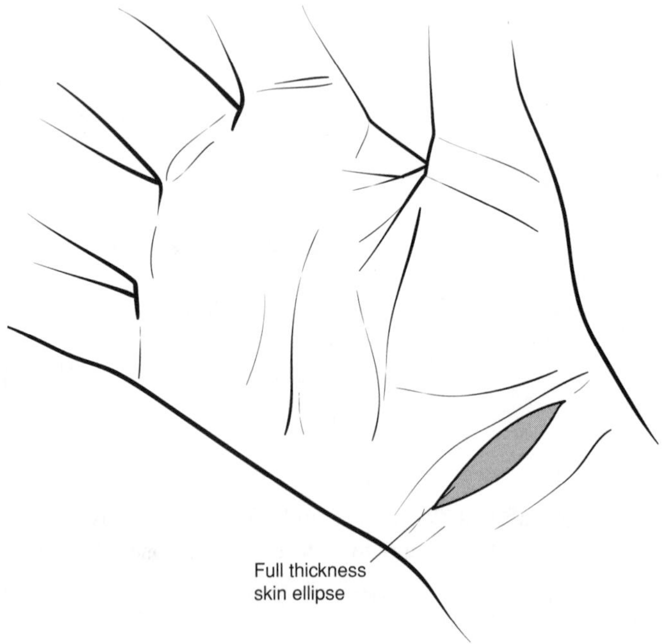

ALTERNATIVE TREATMENTS

- primary healing by contraction and epithelialization
- split-thickness skin graft

SURGICAL ANATOMY

Incision

- tangential, excising 1–2-mm-thick grafts of epidermis and dermis

APPROACHES

Surgical Techniques

- raise a wheel of skin with lidocaine (thickened skin allows for a more tangential cut)
- excise 1–2-mm-thick graft with a skin hook and no. 15 blade
- debride recipient bed of granulation tissue and necrotric debris
- suture edges of graft at recipient bed or wound edge
- apply scarlet red or other nonadherent material
- apply compressive dressing or tie down bolus dressing with wet cotton balls

POSTOPERATIVE MANAGEMENT

- remove dressing at 24 hours only if infection or hematoma is suspected; evacuate hematoma, if present
- otherwise, maintain dressing for 7–10 days

REHABILITATION

- motion of operative extremity in 7–10 days

COMPLICATIONS

- infection of donor or recipient site
- hematoma under graft

SELECTED REFERENCES

Green DP, ed. Operative hand surgery. 3rd ed. 1993:1716.
Sabiston DC Jr, ed. Textbook of surgery. 1981:555.

NOTES

SPLIT-THICKNESS SKIN GRAFT

CPT code **15100 split graft for trunk, arms, or legs; first ≤ 100 cm²**

ICD-9 codes **949.3 third-degree burn, unspecified**
879.8 wound, open skin

INDICATIONS

- third-degree burns
- full-thickness skin loss with adequate vascular bed of subcutaneous tissue, muscle, or periosteum

ALTERNATIVE TREATMENTS

- healing by contraction and epithelialization
- full-thickness skin graft: less contraction but less viable
- pedicle or myocutaneous flap closure

SURGICAL ANATOMY

- preferred donor sites are in areas that can be easily cared for: lateral and anterior thigh (avoid if limb at risk of amputation), buttocks, and lower abdomen

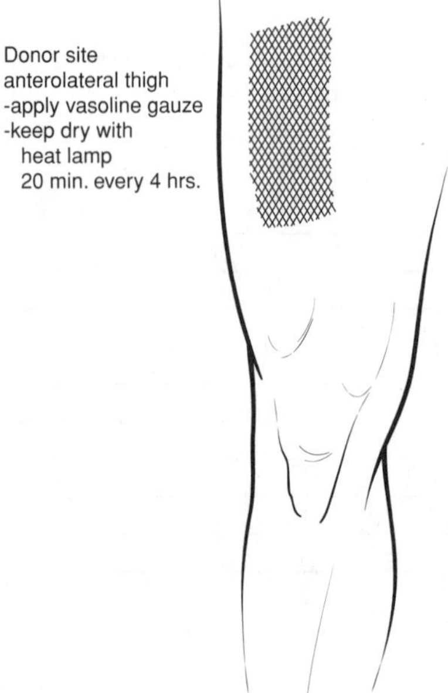

- split-thickness skin grafts are approximately 0.015 inch thick and no thicker than 0.018 inch
- free-hand method with a Goulian knife is technically much more demanding than power dermatomes

Surgical Technique

- debride recipient bed of granulation tissue and necrotic debris
- ensure good capillary bed and hemostasis
- adjust thickness and width of graft on power dermatome
- double-check thickness setting; no. 15 blade should not pass completely through the cutting gap
- lubricate donor site with mineral oil to prevent binding
- assistant holds skin taut with traction using tongue depressor in front of the dermatome
- surgeon applies countertraction behind the dermatome
- advance dermatome slowly and deliberately to prevent skips
- lift dermatome from skin when adequate graft is obtained
- spread graft out evenly, epidermis side up, on mesh card
- use the mesh card with grooves side up or you will make linguini of the graft!
- with the mesh graft, place epidermis side up in the recipient bed
- take care to conform to concave areas and prevent tenting
- suture or staple the graft to the wound edges
- apply nonadherent gauze and then wet cotton balls
- apply compressive dressing and splint the extremity to prevent shearing

POSTOPERATIVE MANAGEMENT

- remove dressing at 24 hours only if infection or hematoma is suspected; evacuate hematoma, if present
- otherwise, maintain dressing for 7–10 days.

REHABILITATION

- motion of operative extremity in 7–10 days.

COMPLICATIONS

- infection of donor or recipient site
- hematoma under graft

SELECTED REFERENCE

Greene DP, ed. Operative hand surgery. 3rd ed. 1993:1711–1739.

MEDIAL GASTROCNEMIUS FLAP

CPT code **15572 formation of direct or tubed pedicle, with or without transfer; scalp, arms, or legs**

ICD-9 code **832.0 open fracture proximal tibia**

INDICATIONS

- soft tissue loss from knee or proximal third of tibia

ALTERNATIVE TREATMENT

- free flap with microvascular anastamosis

SURGICAL ANATOMY

- the vascular pedicle is proximal from the sural artery, which branches from the popliteal artery at the level of the femoral condyle; it enters muscle 3 cm above the joint line

Incision

- Mid-calf, 2 cm behind the posteromedial border of the tibia, curving proximally to the popliteal fossa

APPROACHES

Surgical Technique

- position: supine, limb externally rotated, knee flexed
- deep fascia incised in line with skin incision
- avoid injury to the saphenous vein and nerve
- develop plane between the soleus and gastrocnemius
- dissect sural nerve free and retract posteriorly
- identify median raphe between the medial and lateral heads
- divide the medial head at the achilles tendon
- develop the flap distal to the proximal separating heads at the raphe
- preserve the sural vessel pedicle to the flap
- divide the motor nerve to the flap
- pass deep under the pes anserinus to the anterior skin defect
- can increase arc of rotation by dividing the muscle origin
- place split-thickness skin graft over the muscle

POSTOPERATIVE MANAGEMENT

- splint extremity, limited ambulation
- maintain elevation at level of heart

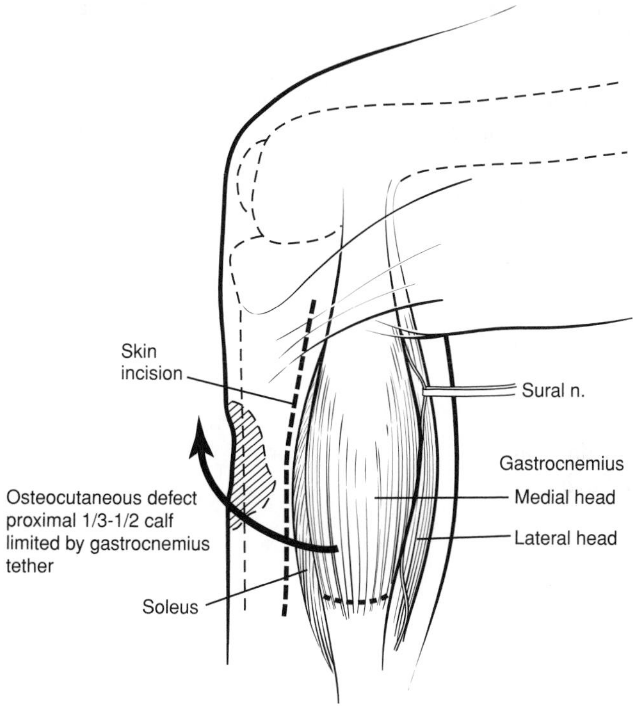

REHABILITATION

- start knee range of motion at 2 weeks

COMPLICATIONS

- graft failure, injury or tension of pedicle
- infection or osteomyelitis

SELECTED REFERENCES

Vos GD, Buehler MJ. Lower extremity local flaps. J Am Acad Orthop Surg 1994;2:342–351.

Masquelet AC. An atlas of flaps of the muscular skeletal system. London: Blackwell Science, 2001.

NOTES

EXCISION, SACRAL PRESSURE ULCER

CPT code **15936 excision, sacral pressure ulcer, in preparation for muscle or myocutaneous flap or skin graft closure**

ICD-9 code **707.0 decubitus ulcer**

INDICATIONS

- sacral decubitis
- severely contaminated sacral decubitis

ALTERNATIVE TREATMENTS

- wet to dry dressings
- whirlpool therapy

SURGICAL ANATOMY

- Gluteus maximus myocutaneous flap preferred for closure

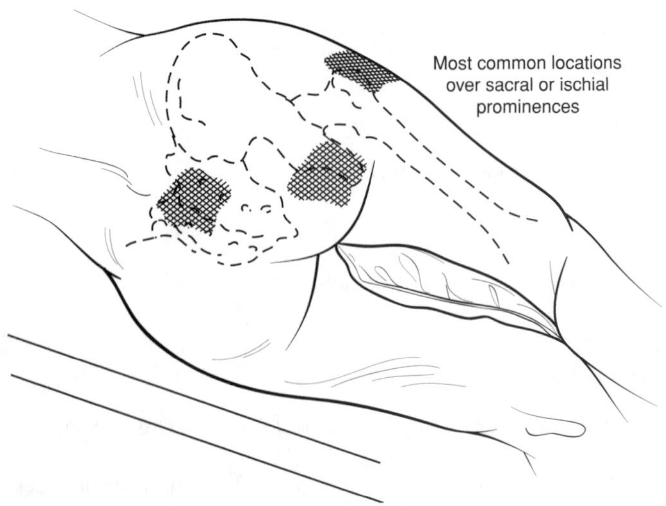

APPROACHES

Surgical Techniques

- debride wound edges to viable bleeding skin
- debride bone from sacrum, if necrotic
- avoid sacral nerve roots

- do not penetrate the cortex into the sacral plexus
- hemostasis, betadine dressing

POSTOPERATIVE MANAGEMENT

- clinitron or low air-loss bed
- strict avoidance of pressure at operative site

REHABILITATION

- collaboration with physiatry is essential
- use of proper seating (or modification of existing wheelchair or bed) is essential
- maximum duration of rest on affected area should be 2 hours before and after healing to prevent recurrent skin breakdown

COMPLICATIONS

- hemorrhage
- sacral nerve injury (may not be an issue in paraplegia)
- osteomyelitis

SELECTED REFERENCE

Grabb WC, Smith WL, Aston SJ et al. Grabb and Smith's Plastic Surgery. Philadelphia: Lippincott-Raven, 1997.

NOTES

JOINT ASPIRATION

CPT code **20610 arthrocentesis, aspiration and/or injection; major joint or bursa (eg, shoulder, hip, knee joint, subacromial bursa)**

ICD-9 codes
716.9 arthropathy, unspecified
711 arthropathy associated with infections
714.0 rheumatoid arthritis
715.1 osteoarthrosis, localized

INDICATIONS

- suspected inflammatory or septic arthritis
- painful hemarthrosis of the knee

ALTERNATIVE TREATMENTS

- incison and drainage

SURGICAL ANATOMY

Aspiration Sites

- shoulder: below the coracoid, just medial to the humeral head (see p. 28–29)
- hip: fluoroscopically guided: anterior to femoral head

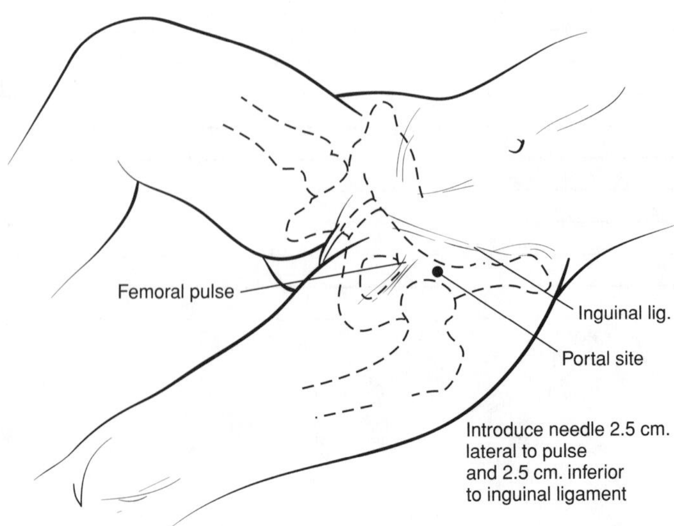

- knee: under the patella, transversely from the lateral border

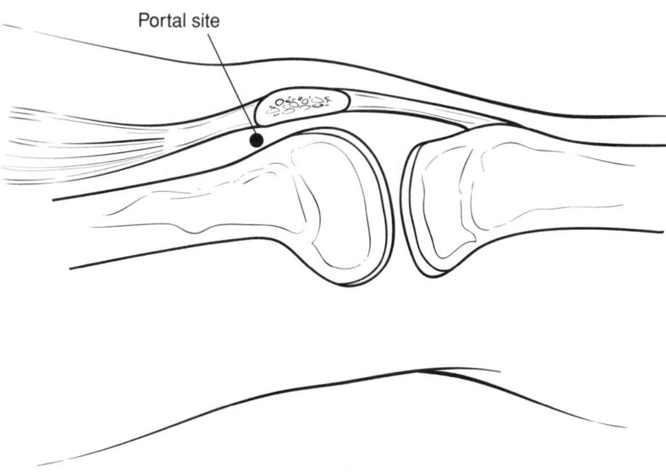

- ankle: between the medial malleolus and the anterior tibial tendon

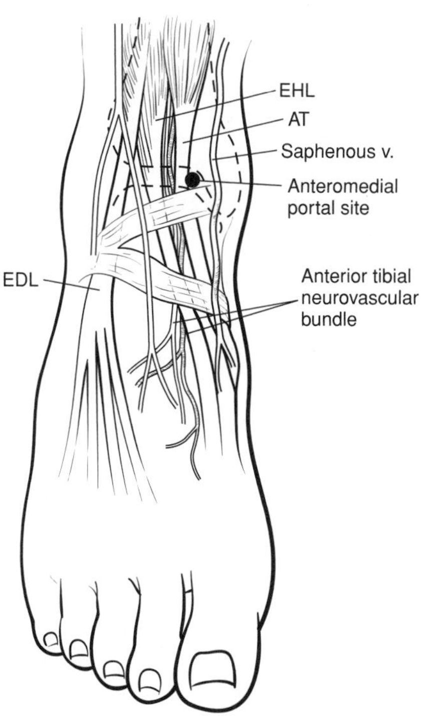

APPROACHES

- site dependent, as shown in illustrations

Surgical Techniques

- prepare site well with betadine and fenestrated drape
- sterile gloves and technique
- aspirate with 18-gauge needle (if necessary)
- take care not to injure cartilage
- for large effusion, hold needle in the joint with hemastat and change the syringe

POSTOPERATIVE MANAGEMENT

- compressive dressing and splint
- synovial analysis: cell count (in tube with anticoagulant), gram stain, culture, or crystal analysis; consider glucose and protein levels
- consider open or arthroscopic debridement, if septic:
  - bacteria on gram stain
  - 50,000 white blood cell count/mL, predominantly polys (PMNs)—cell count is not absolute indication

REHABILITATION

- early motion after incision and debridement

COMPLICATIONS

- joint sepsis from inoculation
- nerve or vascular injury, especially with multiple attempts

SELECTED REFERENCES

Esterhai JL, Gelb I. Adult septic arthritis. Orthop Clin North Am 1991;22:503–514.

Schumacher HR. Atlas of synovial fluid analysis and crystal identification. Philadelphia: Lea & Febiger, 1991.

Sucato DJ, Schwend RM, Gillespie R. Septic arthritis of the hip in children. J Am Acad Orthop Surg 1997;5:249–260.

NOTES

SHOULDER, SELECTIVE INJECTION

CPT code **20610 arthrocentesis, aspiration, and/or injection; major joint or bursa (e.g., shoulder, hip, knee joint, and subacromial bursa)**

ICD-9 codes **726.19 subacromial bursitis**
715.11 osteoarthrosis, localized, shoulder

INDICATIONS

- suspected subacromial impingement: positive Neer's or Hawkins' sign, supraspinatus weakness
- suspected symptomatic acromioclavicular (AC) joint arthritis: tenderness at AC joint, cross-arm adduction pain

ALTERNATIVE TREATMENTS

- open or arthroscopic subacromial decompression
- open or arthroscopic Mumford procedure

APPROACHES

Intraarticular Anterior Injection

- prepare anterior shoulder with betadine
- 40 mg DepoMedrol in 3 cc 1% Lidocaine and 0.5% Marcaine

Subacromial Injection

- prepare posterior shoulder with betadine
- 40 mg DepoMedrol in 3 mL Lidocaine 1%, no. 22 or 25 needle
- pass posterior to anterior just below the posterior acromion, 2 cm from the lateral border of the acromion

Acromioclavicular Joint Injection

- prepare area over AC joint with betadine
- 40 mg DepoMedrol in 1 mL Lidocaine 1%, no. 22 needle
- insert just distal to the prominence of the distal clavicle and pop through the superior AC joint; can inject only 1–2 mL solution

SURGICAL ANATOMY

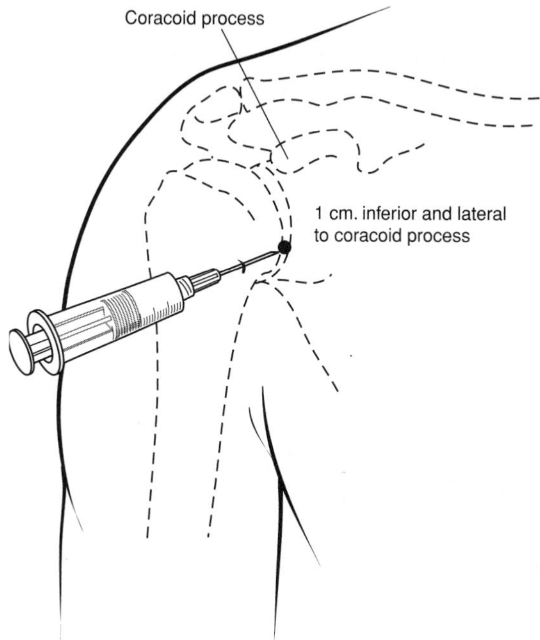

POSTOPERATIVE MANAGEMENT

- re-examine patient; signs of impingement or AC joint arthritis should be improved or eliminated

REHABILITATION

- rotator cuff strengthening exercises for impingement
- physical therapy not effective in isolated AC joint arthritis

COMPLICATIONS

- infection from inoculation
- attritional tear of rotator cuff
- intravascular injection of lidocaine can lead to dizziness, seizure, and even death

SELECTED REFERENCE

See 20610 (p. 24)

GENERAL

INSERTION OF SKELETAL TRACTION

CPT code **20650 insertion of wire or pin with application of skeletal traction, including removal (separate procedure)**

ICD-9 codes
821.01 femur fracture
808.0 acetabular fracture
820.8 femoral neck or hip fracture
812.41 supracondylar humerus fracture
835.01 dislocation of the hip

INDICATIONS

Initial or definitive management with skeletal traction of fractures of the femur or humerus or dislocation of the hip in children or adults

ALTERNATIVE TREATMENTS

- closed reduction, percutaneous pinning of supracondylar fractions
- intramedullary rodding, open reduction–internal fixation, application of external fixation for femur fractures
- open reduction–internal fixation of acetabular fractures

SURGICAL ANATOMY

Incision
- stab wound in the mid-coronal medial distal thigh (avoid Hunter's canal)
- stab wound in the lateral aspect of the tibial tubercle (avoid peroneal nerve)
- stab wound in the medial olecranon (avoid ulnar nerve)

APPROACHES

Surgical Techniques
- position: supine, knee or elbow flexed at 90° (to relax neurovascular structures)
- betadine preparation, with local anesthesia
- longitudinal stab wound <1 cm
- approach distal femur along the metaphysis above the physis, confirm with x-ray as needed; medial to lateral avoids injury to vessels
- approach tibial tubercle laterally and olecranon medially
- using a tibial tubercle pin in a child may cause apophyseal arrest
- insert largest Steinman pin available: 5/64 or 3/32, twist drill
- incise skin on far side, center pin, and cut off excess
- apply traction bow and traction, 7–12 lbs for child's femur
- for a child's femur, use 90–90°; for adult femur, use split Russell
- for a child's elbow, use 90° elbow flexion

POSTOPERATIVE MANAGEMENT

- for a child's femur, apply approximately 3 weeks of traction

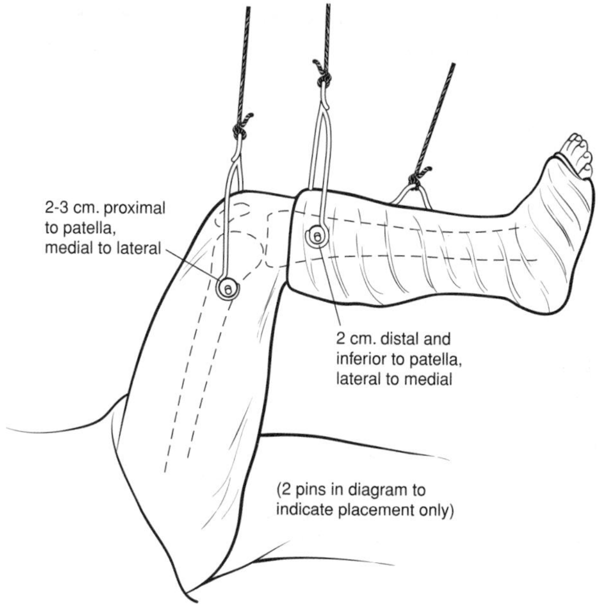

- for a child's elbow, apply 7–10 days of traction
- for the adult hip, apply several weeks of protected weight-bearing

REHABILITATION

- for a child's femur, apply a spica cast for 6–7 weeks and physical therapy with crutches or walker
- for a child's elbow, apply long arm cast for 3 weeks and then start active range of motion
- for the adult hip, apply non-weight-bearing or partial weight-bearing with walker or crutches

COMPLICATIONS

- infection: <1%
- knee stiffness: 2–4%
- injury to neurovascular structure: <1%
- scars
- tibial tubercle apophyseal arrest

SELECTED REFERENCES

Aronson DD, Singer RM, Higgins RF. Skeletal traction for fractures of the femoral shaft in children. J Bone Joint Surg 1987;69A:1435–1439.

Miller PR, Welch MC. The hazards of tibial pin placement in 90-90 skeletal traction. Clin Orthop 1978;135:97–100.

HARDWARE REMOVAL

CPT code **20670** **removal of implant, superficial (e.g., buried wire, pin, or rod; separate procedure)**

ICD-9 code **829** **fracture of unspecified bones**

INDICATIONS

- Prominent hardware irritating skin
- Fracture should be healed

ALTERNATIVE TREATMENT

- Observation

SURGICAL ANATOMY

Incision

- in general, incise through the existing scar
- hypertrophic or unsightly scar can be revised

APPROACHES

Surgical Techniques

- limit size of incision to identify the end of the pin or wire
- sharp dissection to tip of the implant
- grasp the end of the implant with heavy needle driver and pull
- irrigate, close primarily

POSTOPERATIVE MANAGEMENT

- Suture removal in 7–10 days

REHABILITATION

- Early mobilization of extremity

COMPLICATIONS

- Infection
- scar neuroma masquerading as hardware tenderness

NOTES

APPLICATION OF EXTERNAL FIXATOR

CPT code **20690 application of a uniplane (pins or wires in one plane), unilateral, external fixation system**

ICD-9 codes **808.43 multiple pelvic fractures with disruption of pelvic circle**
813.41 Colles' fracture, Smith's fracture
823.30 open fracture of shaft of tibia

INDICATION

- stable mid-diaphyseal open fracture
- simple fracture with associated skin lesions, chronic or traumatic
- temporary, e.g., spanning external fixator for a floating knee or elbow pending definitive fixation

ALTERNATIVE TREATMENTS

- skeletal traction
- cast or Robert Jones dressing
- multiplanar fixator necessary for unstable fractures

SURGICAL ANATOMY

- location specific

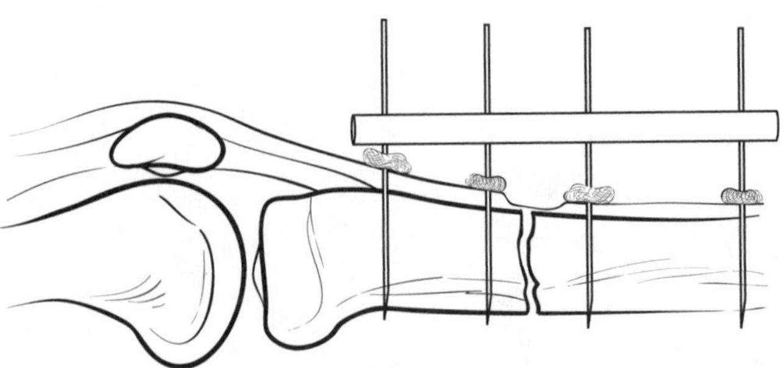

APPROACHES

Surgical Techniques

- tip: with a Synthes tubular fixator, the fracture must be angularly and rotationally aligned before pin placement
- use percutaneous rather than transmuscular approaches, when possible
- avoid placing pins that might compromise care of the open wound, in particular free or rotational flap coverage
- double connecting bar will make construct somewhat more rigid

POSTOPERATIVE MANAGEMENT

- ensure pin site incisions are large enough to prevent pressure or tension on skin edge
- occlusive dressing for 2 days and then
  - half-strength hydrogen peroxide to thoroughly debride pin sites twice daily
  - do not apply bacitracin or other occlusive ointments
  - if soft tissue is significant (thigh and pelvis), wrap pins snugly to prevent skin motion around the pin (see diagram)

COMPLICATIONS

- pin tract infections occur in approximately 10% of cases and usually can be treated by increasing the frequency of cleaning and oral Keflex
- grossly loose pins need to be removed or replaced
- ring sequestrum development is unusual with predrilled pins and careful pin site management
- intramuscular rods should not be placed through a prior pin site if the pin has been in place >10 days

SELECTED REFERENCES

Iannacone WM, Taffat R, Delong WG, et al. Early exchange intra-medullary nailing of distal femoral fractures with vascular injury initially stabilized with external fixation. J Trauma 1994;37:446–451.

Nowotarski PJ, Turen CH, Brumback RJ, et al. Conversion of external fixation to intramedullary nailing for fractures of the shaft of the femur in multiply injured patients. JBJS 2000;82:781–788.

NOTES

REMOVAL OF EXTERNAL FIXATOR

CPT code **20694 removal, under anesthesia, of external fixation system**

ICD-9 code(s) **multiple, e.g., 823.3 tibia fracture, shaft, open**

INDICATIONS

External fixators are applied to stabilize fractures with extensive soft tissue injury, unstable joints, and arthrodesis sites. An external fixator can be removed after healing of the fracture or ligament or osteotomy site. Sometimes an external fixator is used for temporary fracture fixation until soft tissue healing allows definitive internal fixation.

SURGICAL ANATOMY

Incision

- no incision is usually necessary

APPROACHES

Surgical Techniques

- remove frame
- clinically test of union (consider fluoroscopy to confirm fracture healing)
- remove pins
- irrigate pin sites with betadine solution
- curet pin sites, if grossly infected
- dry sterile dressing
- possible cast application

POSTOPERATIVE MANAGEMENT

- specific postoperative management depends on injury: fracture, osteotomy, or soft tissue

REHABILITATION

- specific postoperative management depends on injury: fracture, osteotomy, or soft tissue (e.g., short leg cast (SLC) or patellar-tendon bearing cast (PTB) for 1 month for tibia fracture)

COMPLICATIONS

- refracture
- hemorrhage (secondary to vessel erosion when vessels have been tented over a pin)

SELECTED REFERENCES

Mears DC. External skeletal fixation. Baltimore: Williams & Wilkins, 1983:284.

Pollack AN, Ziran BH. Principles of external fixation. In: Browner BD, et al, eds. Skeletal trauma. Philadelphia: WB Saunders, 1998:284.

NOTES

BONE GRAFTING

CPT code **20900 bone graft, any donor area; minor or small (e.g., dowel or button)**

ICD-9 code(s) **multiple, e.g., 733.82 non-union of fracture**

INDICATIONS

- non-union, bone loss (secondary to tumor, cyst, infection, or fracture), bridge joint in arthrodesis
- a dowel or button graft describes an inlay graft used to span a non-union or arthrodesis site

ALTERNATIVE TREATMENTS

- electrical stimulation or ultrasound for delayed or non-union
- allograft cortical or cancellous bone
- synthetic bone substitutes

SURGICAL ANATOMY

Incision

- bone graft can be harvested from multiple sites, e.g., dorsal radius, iliac crest, Gerdys tubercle
- anterior: incision over the anterior subcutaneous border iliac crest (begin 2 cm posterior to anterior superior iliac spine [ASIS] to avoid damaging the lateral femoral cutaneous nerve)

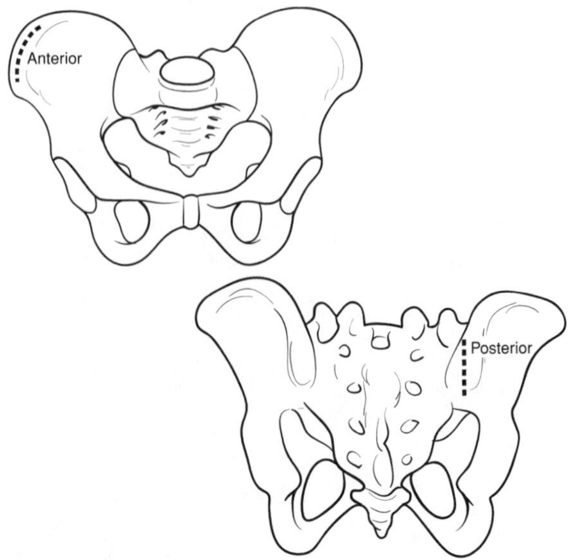

- posterior: vertical and 2 cm lateral to posterior iliac spine

APPROACHES

Surgical Techniques (anterior)

- strip muscles from outer table of the ilium
- strip iliacus from the inner table
- remove crest to harvest cancellous bone (for tricortical graft)
- hemostasis with gelfoam or bone wax
- suction drain placement
- suture periosteum and muscle origin

POSTOPERATIVE MANAGEMENT

Discontinue drain at 24–48 hours

REHABILITATION

- weight-bearing status depends on associated procedures
- pain at bone graft harvest site can persist for several months (warn patient before surgery)

COMPLICATIONS

- hematoma
- infection
- nerve injury (lateral femoral cutaneous nerve)
- muscle hernia
- fracture at bone graft site

SELECTED REFERENCES

Crenshaw AH. Surgical techniques and approaches. In: Canale ST, ed. Campbell's operative orthopaedics. St Louis: Mosby, 1998:40–47.

Kurz LT, Garfin SR, Booth RE. Harvesting autogenous iliac bone grafts: a review of complications and techniques. Spine 1989;14:1324–1331.

NOTES

GENERAL

COMPARTMENT PRESSURE MEASUREMENT

CPT code **20950 monitoring of interstitial fluid pressure (includes insertion of device, e.g., wick catheter technique, needle manometer technique) to detect muscle compartment syndrome**

ICD-9 code **958.8 certain early complications of trauma (compartment syndrome)**

INDICATIONS

- trauma or other muscle injury resulting in severe pain that is out of proportion to apparent injury
- pain with passive muscle stretch and distal palpation
- altered consciousness and any suspicion of elevated pressures (do it–don't wonder)
- occasionally for exercise-induced calf symptoms

ALTERNATIVE TREATMENTS

- immediate fasciotomy
  See CPT 27602 decompressive fasciotomy (p. 206)

TECHNIQUE

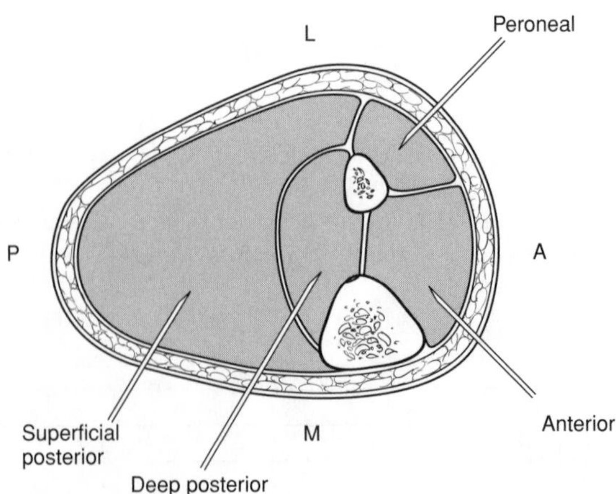

- needle manometer
- wick catheter } follow device instructions
- slit catheter } follow device instructions
- regardless of a particular technique, there are certain principles:
  - ensure lines are flushed with saline
  - place patient supine with the extremity in a normal anatomic position

- introduce needle into mid-portion of compartment; avoid being adjacent to fascia or bone
- zero and calibrate at the level of the site to be tested, *not* at "heart" level
- must check all four compartments in calf

RESULTS

- Consider fasciotomy for
  - pressures >30 mm Hg
  - within 10–30 mm Hg of diastolic pressure

COMPLICATIONS

- nerve or vessel trauma
- increased compartment pressures
- incorrect information

SELECTED REFERENCES

Hargens, AR, Akeson WH, Mubarek SJ, et al. J Orthodp Res 1989;7:902–909.

Matsen FA, Winquist RA, Krugmire RB. Diagnosis and management of compartment syndromes. J Bone Joint Surg Am 1980;62:286

Moed BR, Thorderson PK. Measurement of intracompartmental pressure; a comparison of the slit catheter, side-ported needle, and simple needle. J Bone Joint Surg Am 1993;75:231.

NOTES

PART II

SHOULDER

CLOSED TREATMENT OF VERTEBRAL FRACTURES

CPT code **22310 closed treatment of vertebral body fracture(s), without manipulation, requiring and including casting or bracing**

ICD-9 codes **805.00 cervical spine**
805.2 thoracic spine
805.4 lumbar spine

INDICATIONS

- <50% canal compromise
- <50% loss of vertebral height
- <20º loss of sagittal balance
- no neurologic impairment
- no instability on flexion and extension views
- low risk for non-union

ALTERNATIVE TREATMENTS

- open reduction–internal fixation with posterior instrumentation
- corpectomy and strut graft with anterior instrumentation

Surgical Techniques

- C1 ring: halo vest for Jefferson fractures and displaced lateral mass causing head tilt; otherwise, use two-poster brace
- C2 body: two-poster brace
- C2 odontoid: for type II, use halo vest; for type I or III, use two-poster brace or halo vest
- C2 posterior arch: use two-poster brace for stable type I and halo vest for type II
- C3-C7: Somi or four-poster brace
- T1-T6: thoraco/lumbar/sacral/sacral orthosis (TLSO) with chin bar attachment
- T7-L2: TLSO or three-poster brace
- L3-sacrum: Boston-style LSO or equivalent

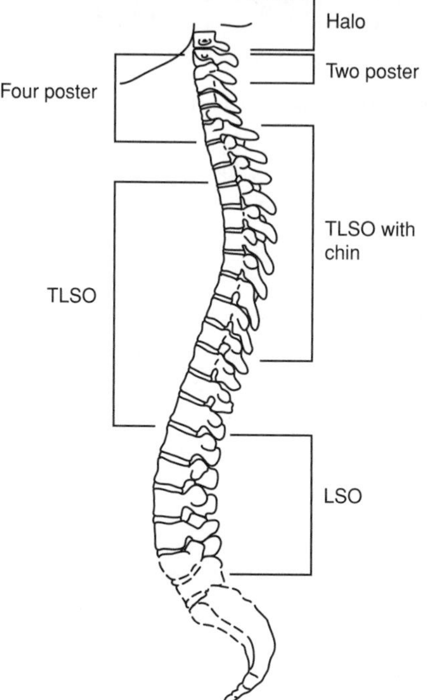

POSTOPERATIVE MANAGEMENT

- initial upright anteroposterior and lateral radiographs in brace
- follow up x-ray in 1 week and then as needed

REHABILITATION

- physical therapy after 12 weeks to restore mobility and function

COMPLICATIONS

- non-union
- loss of coronal or sagittal balance or both
- facet arthropathy, degeneration of motion segments.

SELECTED REFERENCE

Bridwell KH, DeWald RL. The textbook of spinal surgery. New York; Lippincott-Raven, 1991.

SUBACROMIAL BURSECTOMY

SHOULDER

CPT code **23000 removal of subdeltoid bursa**

ICD-9 codes **719.81 calcification of joint, shoulder**
726.11 calcifying tendinitis of shoulder

INDICATIONS

Failure to achieve sustained relief with nonsteroidal anti-inflammatory drugs, physical therapy, modified activity, and subacromial steroid injection. Isolated subacromial bursectomy is rarely indicated with impingement syndrome (need associated acromioplasty).

ALTERNATIVE TREATMENTS

- arthroscopic subacromial bursectomy
- acromioplasty (open or arthroscopic)

SURGICAL ANATOMY

Needle Localization

- directly over calcium deposit
- determined clinically or radiographically

Incision

- lateral deltoid splitting

APPROACHES

Aspiration/Needling Technique

- palpation of skin over tender calcified mass or infiltration
- needle puncture of deposit
- barbotage with syringe or exchange with larger needle
- barbotage with increasing or decreasing needle penetration
- inject corticosteroid

Surgical Techniques

- deltoid splitting incision
- identify raised calcified area on rotator cuff
- curet cavity
- excise affected tissue
- close split in cuff

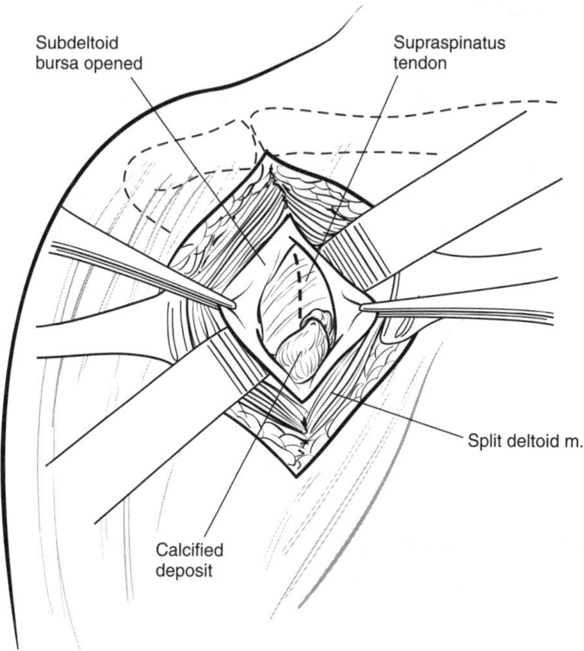

POSTOPERATIVE MANAGEMENT

- sling if using an open approach

REHABILITATION

- pendulum exercises, passive and active range of motion, and return to activity as tolerated

COMPLICATIONS

- infection
- wound hematoma
- axillary nerve injury (with lateral approach) and muscle split >4 cm below acromion

SELECTED REFERENCE

Crenshaw AH. Shoulder and elbow injuries. In Crenshaw AH, ed. Campbell's operative orthopedics. 8th ed. Baltimore: CV Mosby, 1992:1741–1742.

ACROMIOPLASTY

CPT code **23130 acromioplasty or acromionectomy, partial, with or without coracoacromial ligament release**

ICD-9 codes **726.10 disorders of bursae and tendons in shoulder region**
719.41 pain in joint involving shoulder region

INDICATIONS

Well-defined subacromial pain associated with positive impingement tests, a radiographic subacromial bone spur, relief with a subacromial anesthetic injection, and nonresponsive to a well-structured program of physical therapy that includes rotator cuff strengthening.

ALTERNATIVE TREATMENTS

- Subacromial injections of corticosteroid (no more than three); this is usually a temporizing measure and not definitive in many cases.
- Open acromioplasty

SURGICAL ANATOMY

The acromion articulates with the clavicle medially. It is generally best to avoid coplaning the under side of the distal clavicle (to avoid resecting the clavicle and acromion) unless the surgeon plans to do a formal resection of the distal clavicle (Mumford's procedure) as a separate procedure for acromioclavicular arthritis. Coplaning can destabilize the distal clavicle.

Incision

There are two arthroscopic portals: (1) at the "soft spot" posteriorly at the glenohumeral joint line about two finger breadths below the scapular spine; (2) just below the acromion at its lateral border and about one fingerbreadth behind the anterolateral acromion.

APPROACH

- aim for the subacromial space with the obturator

Surgical Techniques

After a complete subacromial bursa resection with a rotary resector, the surgeon identifies the anterolateral corner of the acromion and resects the spur there and establishes the proper depth for further resection. This is best accomplished looking from the posterior portal and resecting with an acromionizer (burr) from the lateral portal.

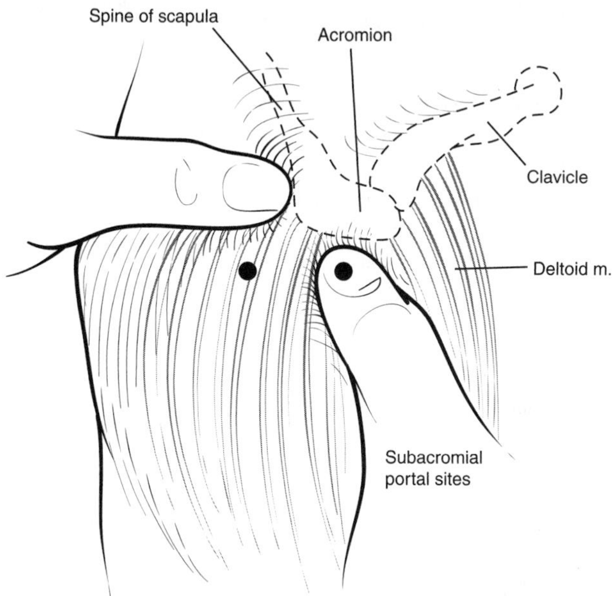

The instuments are then switched, so that the acromionizer is introduced from the posterior portal. The surgeon then uses the flat surface of the posterior acromial undersurface to remove bone in a consistent manner from posterior to anterior, planing down the anterior acromion all the way to and including its anterior edge.

POSTOPERATIVE MANAGEMENT

Use a sling for comfort but start pendulum exercises right away and range of motion as tolerated and then progress to strengthening as tolerated.

REHABILITATION

- progresses rapidly, as noted above

COMPLICATIONS

- These are uncommon; hematoma can limit motion so rarely an aspiration may be necessary
- stiffness is the most likely problem, but this is rare and is best avoided by well-structured physical therapy
- infection is very rare
- coplaning, as described above, can cause acromioclavicular instability

SELECTED REFERENCE

Hawkins R, Bell R, Lippitt S. Atlas of shoulder surgery. St Louis: Mosby, 1996.

REMOVAL OF IMPLANT, SHOULDER

CPT code **23331 removal of foreign body, shoulder, deep (e.g., Neer's hemiarthroplasty removal)**

ICD-9 codes
996.4 hardware complication, other
996.66 infected prosthesis
996.67 infected hardware

INDICATIONS

- infected prosthesis or hardware
- broken or displaced prosthesis or hardware
- inadvertent foreign body

ALTERNATIVE TREATMENTS

- suppression antibiotic therapy
- retain foreign body

APPROACHES

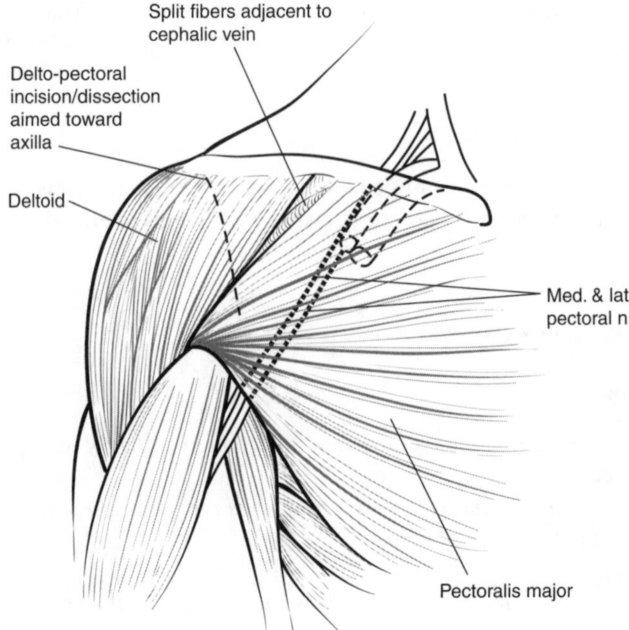

- deltopectoral (for hemiarthroplasty)
- lateral deltoid splitting (for intramedullary rods, screws or tension bands)

Surgical Technique

- position: beach chair
- incision: coracoid to mid-arm (deltopectoral)
- blunt dissection between deltoid and pectoralis
- cephalic vein retracted medially or laterally
- subscapularis taken off medial to lesser tuberosity
- capsule taken with the subscapularis or separately
- component(s) removed
- *all* cement and devitalized tissue removed, if infected
- debridement
- irrigation
- closure with drainage

POSTOPERATIVE MANAGEMENT

- antibiotics as indicated
- sling and swath immobilization

REHABILITATION

- immediate motion of the elbow, wrist, or hand
- shoulder motion as indicated

COMPLICATIONS

- recurrent infection
- fracture non-union or malunion
- subscapularis detachment

NOTES

RUPTURE, LONG HEAD OF BICEPS

SHOULDER

CPT code	**23430 tenodesis of long tendon of biceps**
ICD-9 codes	**727.62 tendons of biceps (long head)**
	726.12 bicipital tenosynovitis

INDICATIONS

- rupture of long head of biceps
- chronic tendinosis with pain
- cosmetic deformity associated with rupture (and associated weakness)

ALTERNATIVE TREATMENTS

- nonsteroidal anti-inflammatory drugs, heat or ice, gentle range of motion exercises
- use of ultrasound or iontophoresis
- may not be required in elderly or infirm patients with restricted activities of daily living

SURGICAL ANATOMY

- anterior approach
- incision with the deltopectoral approach, beginning 2 cm distal to the coracoid process
- internervous plane between deltoid (axillary) and pectoralis major (medial and lateral pectoral) muscles

Surgical Techniques

- historically, the "keyhole" technique was used to insert the proximal tendon stump into the bicipital groove via drillhole (illustrated)
- today, the suture is anchored into the bicipital groove with a multiple suture anchor technique

POSTOPERATIVE MANAGEMENT

- immobilize elbow in flexion to rest for 10–14 days

REHABILITATION

- begin active or gravity-assisted range of motion after 3 weeks
- begin isotonic or isokinetic strengthening after 6 weeks

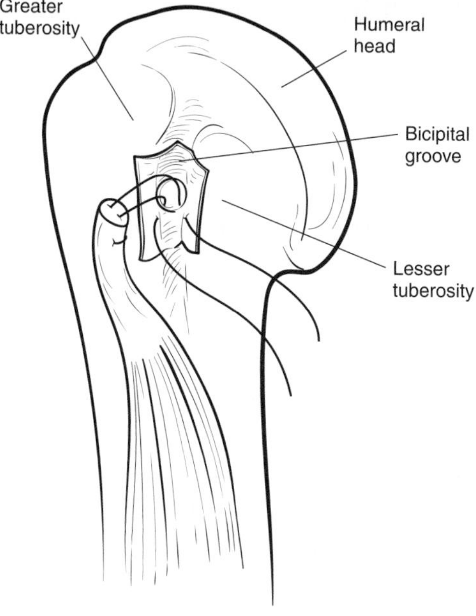

COMPLICATIONS

- rerupture (rare)
- may result in decompensation of rotator cuff function, especially for overhead activities and throwing

SELECTED REFERENCE

Justis EJ. In Crenshaw AH, ed. Campbell's operative orthopaedics. 7th ed. St Louis: Mosby, 1987:2237–2239.

NOTES

ANTERIOR STABILIZATION, SHOULDER

CPT code **23450 capsulorrhaphy, anterior; Putti-Platt procedure or Magnuson-type operation**

ICD-9 codes **718.31 recurrent dislocation of shoulder joint**
718.21 pathologic dislocation of shoulder joint
905.7 late effect of sprain and strain (subluxation)

INDICATIONS

- recurrent anterior dislocation or subluxation of shoulder
- recurrent "drop attacks" (subluxation)
- usually in patients younger than 30 years at time of first dislocation

ALTERNATIVE TREATMENTS

- continued conservative treatment; avoid abduction and external rotation
- arthroscopic Bankhart repair

SURGICAL ANATOMY

- use the deltopectoral approach by keeping an internervous plane between the deltoid (axillary) and pectoralis major (medial and lateral pectoral) muscles
- gently medially retract the short head of biceps and coracobrachialis (musculocutaneous nerve)
- incise the subscapularis transversely to its fibers, approximately 1 cm medial to its insertion to assist in repair

Surgical Techniques

- Putti-Platt: imbrication of the subscapularis to prevent external rotation
- Magnuson-Stack: advance the capsule and subscapularis into trough in the humerus lateral to the bicipital groove in the greater tuberosity
- Bristow: transect the corocoid process with attached conjoined tendon (short head biceps and coracobrachialis); fix with screw medial and inferior to capsule to buttress against recurrent subluxation

POSTOPERATIVE MANAGEMENT

- maintain in sling and swath to avoid abduction and external rotation of shoulder for 3–4 weeks (6 weeks for Bristow bone healing)

REHABILITATION

- begin Codman (pendulum) exercises at 10–14 days
- begin overhead and strengthing exercises including internal and external rotation isotonic strengthening at 5–6 weeks

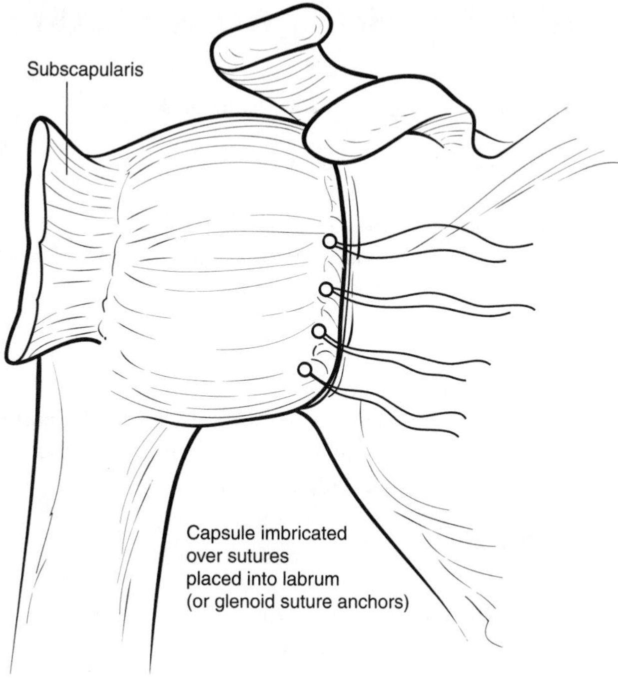

COMPLICATIONS

- injury to the axillary (too inferior dissection) or musculocutaneous (too far medial dissection) nerves
- recurrent dislocation (occurs <6%)
- loss of external rotation and compromise of some sporting activities (throwing and hockey)
- possible development of osteoarthritis if repair is too tight and joint is overloaded

SELECTED REFERENCE

Freeman BL. In Crenshaw AH, ed. Campbell's operative orthopaedics. 7th ed. St Louis: Mosby, 1987:2187–2205.

NOTES

GLENOHUMERAL HEMIARTHROPLASTY

CPT code **23470 arthroplasty, glenohumeral joint, hemiarthroplasty**

ICD-9 codes **715.11 osteoarthrosis, localized, primary**
812.02 anatomic neck fracture with displacement
733.41 osteonecrosis, head of humerus
714.0 rheumatoid arthritis (with rotator cuff pathology)

INDICATIONS

- four-part fracture of the proximal humerus with anatomic neck involvement and high likelihood of osteonecrosis or non-union
- osteoarthritis or rheumatoid arthritis with significant rotator cuff pathology or glenoid deficiency are contraindications to use of glenoid component (expect pain relief without significantly improved motion)

ALTERNATIVE TREATMENT(S)

- fracture
  - open reduction-internal fixation in young patient
  - resection in elderly, debilitated patient
- arthritis
  - conservative therapy including nonsteroidal anti-inflammatory drugs, heat, activity modification
  - total shoulder arthroplasty

SURGICAL ANATOMY

- use the deltopectoral approach by keeping an internervous plane between the deltoid (axillary) and pectoralis major (medial and lateral pectoral) muscles
- gently medially retract the short head of biceps and coracobrachialis (musculocutaneous nerve)

APPROACHES

- surgical approach via the anterior deltopectoral incision
- identify and protect the cephalic vein
- incise subscapularis and capsule as one layer just medial to the bicipital groove and reflect medially
- average 30° of retroversion of component
- soft tissue balancing is critical
  - avoid excessive laxity or "overstuffing"
  - approximately 50% anteroposterior translation of component is appropriate
  - test especially in external rotation
- use third-generation cementing technique: canal lavage, vacuum mixing, and pressurization

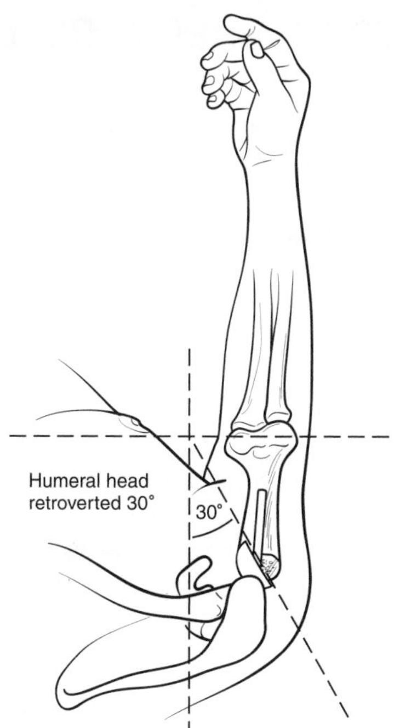

POSTOPERATIVE MANAGEMENT

- pain control usually is not difficult
- dry sterile dressing until wound is dry

REHABILITATION

- use three-stage Neer's rehabilitation protocol
- begin Codman's exercises after 10–14 days (avoid external rotation)
- begin isotonic strengthening at 6 weeks

COMPLICATIONS

- avoid "taking down" the deltoid with attendant failure of repair
- limited range of motion due to pre-existing rotator cuff pathology or inadequate rehabilitation
- injury to the axillary or musculocutaneous nerves
- late secondary wear of the glenoid surface

SELECTED REFERENCES

Hoppenfeld S. Physical Examination of the spine and extremities. New York: Appleton-Century-Crofts, 1976.

Neer CS. Shoulder reconstruction. Philadelphia: WB Saunders, 1990.

CLAVICULAR FRACTURES, CLOSED TREATMENT

CPT codes **23500 without manipulation**
23505 with manipulation

ICD-9 code **810.02 fracture of clavicle**

MECHANISM OF INJURY

- direct blow or axial load to upper limb

ANATOMIC CONSIDERATIONS

- subcutaneous location makes fractures susceptible to integumentary compromise
- proximity to subclavian vein and brachial plexus leads to occasional neurovascular injury

CLASSIFICATION

- nonstandardized
- medial, mid-shaft, and distal thirds denote location best
- relation to coracoclavicular and acromioclavicular ligaments denotes displacement patterns

ASSESSMENT

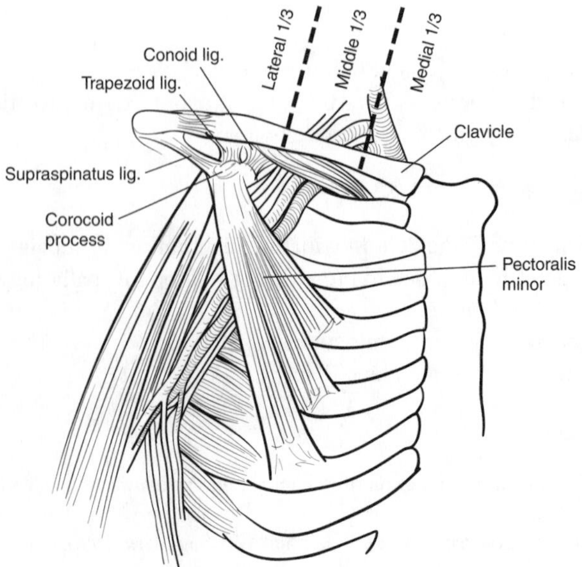

- injury patterns reflect mechanism of loadings
- associated shoulder, C-spine, and chest injuries need to be assessed
- swelling, deformity, and pseudopalsy of shoulder are common
- radiographs should include anteroposterior, 20° cranial caudal views
- computed tomography is helpful in medial or sternoclavicular injuries

MANAGEMENT

- emergent treatment is "first aid": splinting with ice and rest
- definitive treatment consists of modified immobilization (sling, figure-of-eight) until functional recovery
- by 10–21 days, range of movement is increased according to pain tolerance, avoiding weight-bearing
- isometrics for 6 weeks and then resistance exercises
- operative treatment may be warranted for open fracture, neurovascular injury, potential skin compromise, bilateral fractures, unstable "floating" shoulder with associated scapular injury, flail chest or nonunion.

COMPLICATIONS

Internal rotation with "scapular" winging, cosmetic deformity, neurovascular (NV) compromise, decreased range of motion or strength, and nonunion are possible with nonoperative treatment.

NOTES

CLOSED TREATMENT OF ACROMIOCLAVICULAR JOINT DISLOCATION

CPT code **23545 closed treatment of acromioclavicular dislocation, with manipulation**

ICD-9 code **831.04 closed dislocation of acromioclavicular (joint)**

INDICATIONS

- types I and II: closed treatment
- type III: probably closed treatment but controversial
- types IV, V, and VI: open reduction–internal fixation

ALTERNATIVE TREATMENTS

- type III: open reduction–internal fixation in one who performs heavy lifting

SURGICAL ANATOMY

- type I: intact acromioclavicular (A-C) ligaments
- type II: A-C ligaments completely torn and coracoclavicular ligament intact
- type III: A-C and coracoclavicular (CC) ligaments torn
- type IV: clavicle displaced into trapezius
- type V: severe vertical separation from scapula
- type VI: clavicle displaced inferiorly to acromion or coracoid (rare)

APPROACHES

- Kenny Howard brace (illustrated)
- “skillful neglect”

REHABILITATION

- rest or pain control for 2–4 days
- begin range of movement and strength exercises after 4 days and progress as tolerated

COMPLICATIONS

- acute brachial plexus or vascular injury
- weakness
- chronic pain
- chronic deformity
- skin compromise in brace

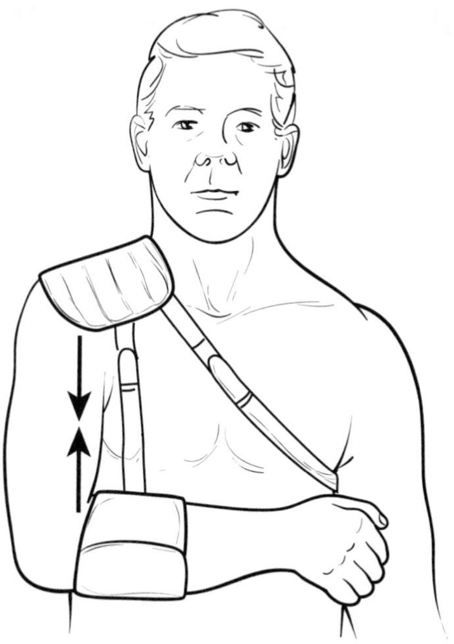

SELECTED REFERENCES

Nuber GW, Bowen MK. Acromioclavicular joint injuries and distal clavicle fractures. J Am Acad Orthop Surg 1997;5:11–18.

Rockwood CS, Green DR, Bucholz RW, Heckman J. Fractures in adults. 4th ed. Philadelphia: Lippincott, 1996.

NOTES

TREATMENT SURGICAL NECK FRACTURE, HUMERUS

CPT code **23605 closed treatment of proximal humeral (surgical or anatomical neck) fracture, with manipulation, with or without skeletal traction**
23615 open treatment of proximal humeral fracture

ICD-9 code **812.01 closed fracture of surgical neck, humerus**

INDICATIONS

Overall goal of care is to preserve function. Minimally displaced fractures can be treated closed. Displaced fractures (anatomic head >40°, shaft fragments >2 cm, or tuberosities >1 cm) should be repaired.

In low demand patients up to 80% displacement and 60° angulation can be tolerated if bone in apposition.

ALTERNATIVE TREATMENTS

- percutaneous Steinman pins
- tension band
- cannulated screws
- plate and screws
- intramedullary fixation (locked or with tension band)
- hemiarthroplasty

SURGICAL ANATOMY

- supraspinatus attaches to greater tuberosity
- subscapularis attaches to lesser tuberosity
- angle of anatomic neck varies but radiographs of the contralateral side can be helpful

Incision

- deltopectoral: incise coracoid to deltoid tubercle
- deltoid splitting: lateral acromion distal, not to exceed 4 cm

APPROACHES

Surgical Techniques

Be sure the patient is positioned to obtain radiographic control. Attempt closed manipulation before preparation and drape because 20% of patients can be

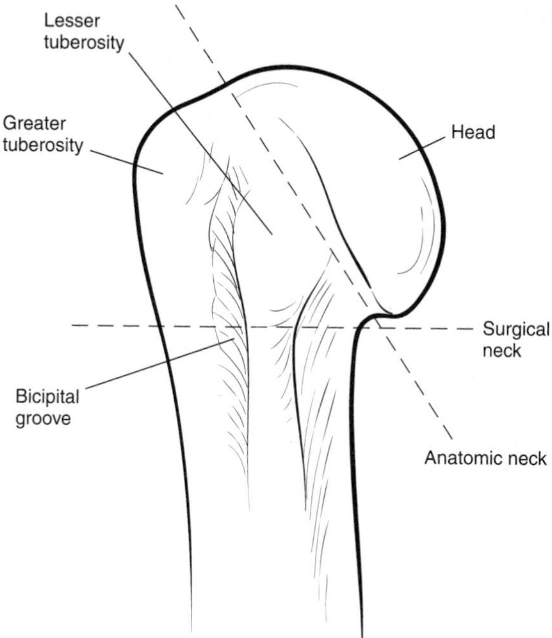

treated with closed reduction. Whenever possible, use minimally invasive techniques. Open reduction should focus on re-establishing normal relations between tendon lengths and bony antomy without injuring arterial supply.

POSTOPERATIVE MANAGEMENT

- sling: encourage immediately range of motion at elbow and digits

REHABILITATION

- gentle pendulum and Codman exercises at 7–10 days
- isometric exercises at 3 weeks and active range of motion with gentle resistance at 6 weeks

COMPLICATIONS

- implant malposition
- non-union or malunion
- avascular necrosis (primarily with attempted anatomic neck repair)
- arthrofibrosis
- nerve lesions (deltoid and muscular cutaneous)
- infection

SELECTED REFERENCES

Bigliani LU. Fractures of the proximal humerus. In: Rockwood CA, Matsen FA, eds. The shoulder. Philadelphia: WB Saunders, 1990.

Burstein AH. Fracture classification systems: do they work and are they useful? JBJS Am 1993;75:1743–1744.

Gerber C, Scheinberger AG, Vin H. The arterial vascularization of the humeral head. J Bone Joint Surg 1990;72:1486–1494.

Koval KJ, Gallagher MA, Marsicano JG, et al. Functional outcome after minimally displaced fractures of the proximal part to the humerus. J Bone Joint Surg Am 1997;79:203.

Kristiansen B, Angerman P, Larsen TK. Functional results following fractures of the proximal humerus. Arch Orthop Trauma Surg 1989;108:339.

Szyszkowitz R, Seggl W, Schleifer P, Cundy PJ. Proximal humeral fractures. Management techniques & expected results. Clin Orthop 1993;292:13–25.

Rockwood CS, Green DP, Bucholz RW, Heckman J. Fractures in adults. 4th ed. Philadelphia: Lippincott, 1996.

NOTES

PART III

ELBOW

EXCISION OLECRANON BURSA

CPT code	**24105**	**excision, olecranon bursa**
ICD-9 codes	**726.33**	**olecranon bursitis**
	714.0	**rheumatoid arthritis**
	274.82	**gouty tophi of other sites**
	727.3	**other bursitis disorders**

INDICATIONS

- failure of conservative treatment including cushioned relief splinting with elbow pad and sterile aspirations with or without steroid injections
- open draining wounds from gout, rheumatoid arthritis, or purulent bursitis

ALTERNATIVE TREATMENTS

- prolonged cushioned relief splinting
- aspiration with or without steroid injections

SURGICAL ANATOMY

Incision
- posterior
- posterolateral (illustrated)

APPROACHES

Surgical Techniques
- supine
- arm over chest
- brachial tourniquet
- thin skin incision
- attempt bursectomy in situ
- excise open skin edges to healthy skin
- meticulous hemostasis
- closure over drain
- compressive dressing with elbow flexed 90º

POSTOPERATIVE MANAGEMENT

- initial postoperative dressing for 7–10 days with immobilization
- gradual mobilization

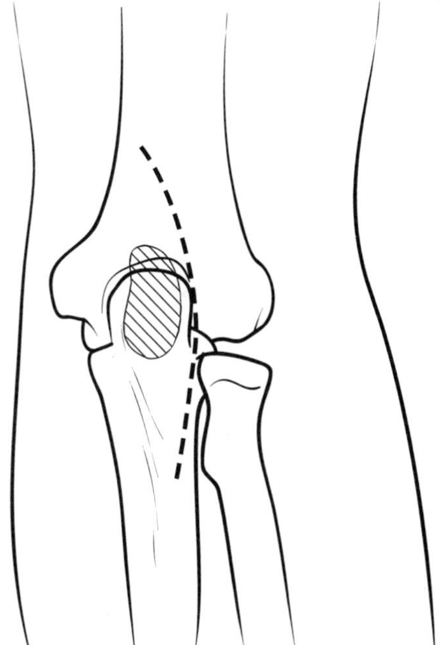

REHABILITATION

- cushioned relief splint for 1–2 months
- avoid direct blows to olecranon

COMPLICATIONS

- postoperative hematoma
- recurrence

SELECTED REFERENCES

Canoso JJ. Idiopathic or traumatic olecranon bursitis. Clinical features and bursal fluid analysis. Arthritis Rheum 1977;20:1213.

Stewart NJ, Manzanares JB, Morrey BF. Surgical treatment of aseptic olecranon bursitis. J Shoulder Elbow Surg 1997;6:49–53.

NOTES

EXCISION RADIAL HEAD

CPT code **24130 excision, radial head**

ICD-9 codes
813.05 radial head fracture
813.06 radial neck fracture
714.06 rheumatoid arthritis
733.81 malunion of fracture
715.13 primary localized osteoarthosis

INDICATIONS

- severe fracture comminution that cannot be reconstructed
- malunion with pain and limited forearm rotation or elbow motion
- part of elbow synovectomy with rheumatoid arthritis/hemophilic arthroplasty

ALTERNATIVE TREATMENTS

- open reduction–internal fixation of acute fracture
- metallic implant arthroplasty (indicated with associated valgus instability, proximal migration of the radius, or a posterior ulnohumeral instability with coronoid fracture)
- arthroscopic synovectomy without radial head resection

SURGICAL ANATOMY

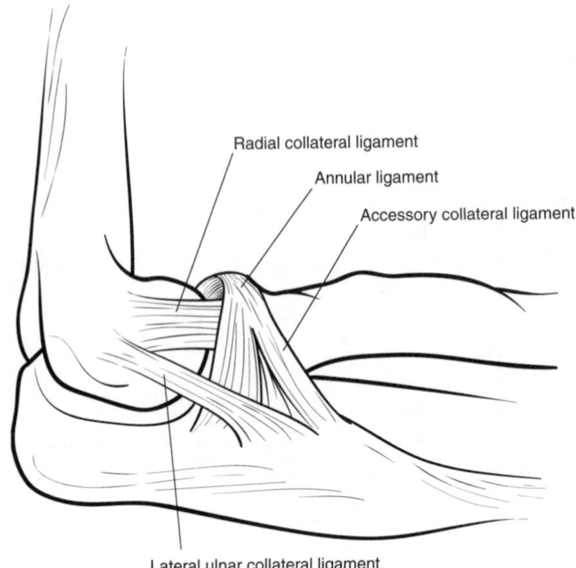

APPROACHES

- lateral: Kaplan (ECRL/EDC)
- posterolateral: Kocher (ECU/anconeus)

Surgical Techniques

- supine
- hand table
- brachial tourniquet
- full-thickness flaps for visualization of muscle intervals
- avoid injury to radial nerve from distal dissection
- protect lateral ulnohumeral ligament complex from lateral epicondyle to crista supinatoris (posterior side of the ulna at the proximal radioulnar joint)
- excise enough head so that the lesser sigmoid notch (ulnar articular surface of proximal radioulnar joint) is fully visible
- imbricate capsule/lateral ligament complex to avoid posterolateral rotatory instability

POSTOPERATIVE MANAGEMENT

- splint 90° until initial dressing change at approximately 1 week
- with posterolateral rotational instability (PLRI) and imbricated or repaired lateral ligament complex, also splint in full pronation

REHABILITATION

- active assisted and passive range of motion with preoperative contracture
- progress with activities as tolerated once wound heals
- if lateral ligament complex has been repaired or reconstructed, protect it by allowing flexion and extension with the forearm in full pronation

COMPLICATIONS

- symptomatic proximal migration of the radius (with associated Essex-Lopresti lesions)
- valgus instability (with associated medial collateral ligament [MCL] injuries)
- posterior ulnohumeral instability (with associated elbow dislocations and coronoid fractures)
- radial nerve injury

SELECTED REFERENCES

Hotchkiss RN. Displaced fractures of the radial head: internal fixation or excision. J Am Acad Orthop Surg 1997;5:1–10.

Morrey BF, Chao EY, Hui FC. Biomechanical study of the elbow following excision of the radial head. J Bone Joint Surg 1979;61A:63.

REPAIR BICEPS RUPTURE

CPT code **24342** **reinsertion of ruptured biceps or triceps tendon, distal, with or without tendon graft**

ICD-9 codes **727.62** **nontraumatic rupture of tendon of biceps, long head**
841.8 **strain and sprain of other specified sites of elbow and forearm**

INDICATIONS

- ruptured biceps or triceps at elbow

ALTERNATIVE TREATMENTS

- nonoperative treatment (limited supination strength)
- tenodesis to brachialis
- if chronic, reconstruction with fascia lata or hamstring

SURGICAL ANATOMY

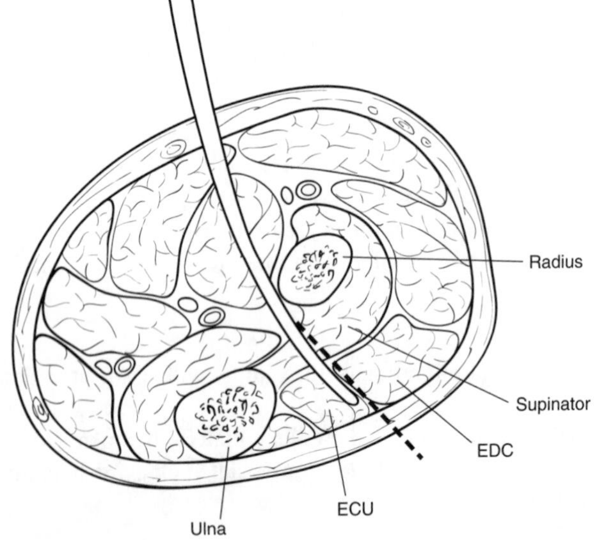

Reproduced from BF Morrey.

APPROACHES

- anterior
  - transverse
  - longitudinal (Henry)
- combined anterior/posterior (Boyd/Anderson)

Surgical Techniques

- supine, hand table
- brachial tourniquet (sterile if chronic or proximal retraction)
- anterior approach
  - FCR/BR interval
  - lateral antebrachial cutaneous nerve
  - leash of Henry
  - radial nerve proper (proximal), superficial sensory branch, and posterior interosseous branch (distal)
  - attach tendon to biceps tuberosity with drill holes or suture anchors
- Boyd/Anderson
  - anterior to find tendon and pass sutures posteriorly or dorsally
  - pass on medial border of radius, not lateral border of ulna (to avoid disrupting the interosseous membrane with risk of synostosis)
  - avoid exposure of ulna, perform muscle splitting instead

POSTOPERATIVE MANAGEMENT

- posterior splint with elbow flexed 90°, neutral forearm rotation
- avoid prolonged immobilization, which could impair functional outcome

REHABILITATION

- with secure repair, begin forearm rotation at 90° flexion within first week postoperatively to avoid synostosis
- protected mobilization without resistance during the first 3 months
- progressive strengthening for next 3 months
- begin full use at 6 months

COMPLICATIONS

- rerupture
- synostosis
- radial nerve palsy
- lateral antebrachial cutaneous nerve neuropraxia

SELECTED REFERENCES

Kelly EW, Morrey BF, O'Driscoll SW. Complications of repair of the distal biceps tendon with the modified two-incision technique. J Bone Joint Surg 2000;82A: 1575–1581.

Strauch RJ, Michelson H, Rosenwasser MP. Repair of rupture of the distal tendon of the biceps brachii. Review of the literature and report of three cases treated with a single anterior incision and suture anchors. Am J Orthop 1997;26:1–6.

TENNIS ELBOW RELEASE

CPT code	**24356**	**fasciotomy, lateral or medial (e.g., tennis elbow or epicondylitis); with partial ostectomy**
ICD-9 codes	**726.32**	**lateral epicondylitis**
	726.31	**medial epicondylitis ("Golfer's elbow")**

INDICATIONS

Failure of conservative management including nonsteroidal anti-inflammatory drugs, counterforce bracing, steroid injection, and therapy

ALTERNATIVE TREATMENTS

- extensor origin detachment or lengthening
- annular or orbicular ligament resection
- anconcus flap for revision

SURGICAL ANATOMY

incision
- lateral
- medial

APPROACHES

Surgical Techniques
- position: supine
- incision: lateral
- incise deep antebrachial fascia
- split common extensor origin to expose ECRB
- debridement of granulation tissue and any avulsed tendon
- tip of lateral epicondyle excised

POSTOPERATIVE MANAGEMENT

- splinting 1–2 weeks

REHABILITATION

- light exercises and isometrics at 4 weeks
- strengthening at 6 weeks
- sports at 2–4 months

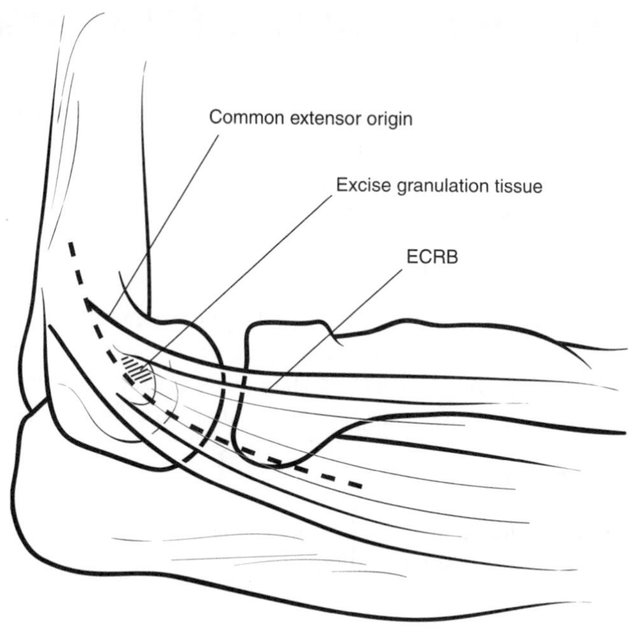

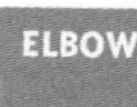

COMPLICATIONS

- failure to relieve symptoms
- iatrogenic nerve injury

SELECTED REFERENCES

Jobe FW, Licotti MG. Lateral and medial epicondylitis. J Am Acad Orthop Surg 1994; 2;1–8.

Nirschl R. Tennis elbow—the surgical treatment of lateral epicondylitis. J Bone Joint Surg 1979:61A:832–839.

NOTES

TREATMENT HUMERAL SHAFT FRACTURE

CPT code **24500 closed treatment of humeral shaft fracture; without manipulation**
24516 open treatment of humeral shaft fracture

ICD-9 code **812.21 closed fracture humeral shaft**

INDICATIONS

Closed treatment suffices for most fractures. Fractures with >20° anterior angulation, >30° varus, or >3 cm shortening can be considered for open reduction–internal fixation. Absolute indications for operative treatment include open fracture, floating elbow, and nerve injury after closed manipulation.

ALTERNATIVE TREATMENTS

- intramedullary rodding: antegrade or retrograde
- open reduction, compression plating

SURGICAL ANATOMY

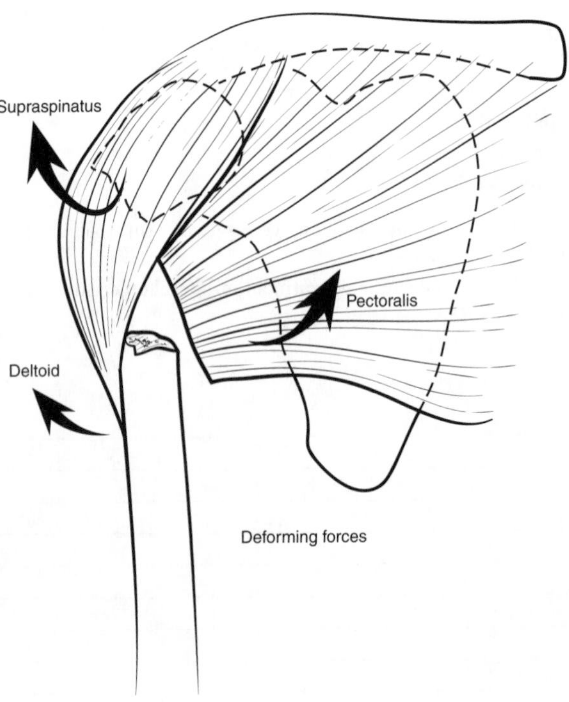

The humeral head and shaft are collinear, whereas the distal humerus flares anteriorly. Proximally the axillary nerve lies with the posterior humeral circumflex artery & vein 5–6 cm distal to the acromion. The radial nerve is relatively fixed at the middle ⅓ of the humeral shaft as it passes laterally through the intermuscular septum.

Incision

- intramedullary nailing: anterior acromial approach, deltoid split or triceps split for retrograde approach
- plating: anterolateral, direct lateral, medial, and posterior

APPROACHES

Surgical Techniques

- humeral plating is currently favored over the intramedullary nail except in weight-bearing situations

POSTOPERATIVE MANAGEMENT

- soft dressing without splint

REHABILITATION

- active and passive range of motion of all associated joints

COMPLICATIONS

- nerve lesions
- non-union or malunion
- painful hardware

SELECTED REFERENCES

Gregory P, Sanders R. Compression plating versus intramedullary fixation of humeral shaft fractures. J Am Acad Orthop Surg 1997;5:215–223.

Sarmiento A, Kinman PB, Galvin EG, et al. Functional bracing of fractures of the shaft of the humerus. J Bone Joint Surg 1977;59:596–601.

NOTES

CLOSED REDUCTION OF ELBOW DISLOCATION

CPT code **24605 treatment of closed elbow dislocation, requiring anesthesia**

ICD-9 codes
832.00 closed unspecified dislocation of elbow
832.02 closed posterior dislocation of elbow
832.10 open unspecified dislocation of elbow
832.12 open posterior dislocation of elbow

INDICATIONS

- elbow dislocation with or without associated fractures (typically of the radial head and coronoid but also consider osteochondral injuries of the capitellum and trochlea)

ALTERNATIVE TREATMENTS

- options are for anesthetic: none, local infiltration, conscious sedation, or general anesthetic
- in pediatric patients, evaluate for pure radiocapitellar dislocation (aka nursemaid's elbow)

SURGICAL ANATOMY

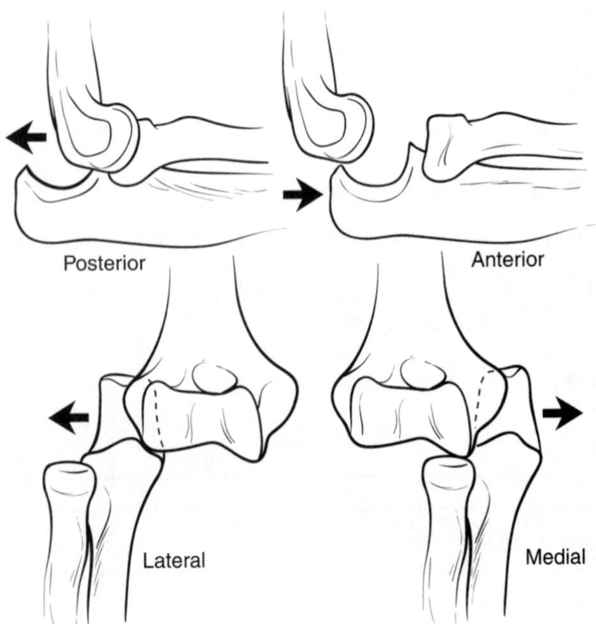

- posterolateral ulnohumeral dislocation (typical)
- posterolateral dislocation progresses from lateral to medial
- medial (rare)
- associated proximal radioulnar diastasis (rare and severe)

APPROACHES

- supine or lateral decubitus

Manipulation Technique

- elbow in 60–90° of flexion
- proximal forearm traction to lift coronoid off of trochlea
- distal axial traction on forearm
- thumb push on olecranon
- reduction clunk usually obvious
- confirm with radiography or fluoroscopy

POSTOPERATIVE MANAGEMENT

- 90–100° splint, neutral forearm rotation
- consider open reduction–internal fixation for associated fractures, especially if unstable

REHABILITATION

- minimize immobilization usually for 1 week for simple dislocations without associated fractures (or with minimal type I radial head and type I coronoid fractures)

COMPLICATIONS

- flexion contracture related to prolonged immobilization (>3 weeks)
- entrapped medial epicondyle (in adolescents nearing skeletal maturity, check comparison views)
- entrapped median nerve: Matev's sign (perform neurologic examination pre- and postreduction)
- recurrent instability, specifically posterolateral rotatory instability

SELECTED REFERENCES

Josefsson PO, Gentz CF, Johnell O, et al. Surgical versus nonsurgical treatment of ligamentous injuries following dislocation of the elbow joint. A prospective randomized study. J Bone Joint Surg 1987;69A:605.

O'Driscoll SW, Morrey BF, Korinek S, An K. Elbow subluxation and dislocation: a spectrum of instability. Clin Orthop 1992;280:186.

CLOSED REDUCTION OF NURSEMAID'S ELBOW

CPT code **24640 closed treatment of radial head subluxation in child, nursemaid's elbow, with manipulation**

ICD-9 codes **832.01 closed anterior elbow dislocation**

INDICATIONS

- acute limitation in forearm rotation and elbow motion after a traction-type injury in a young child

ALTERNATIVE TREATMENTS

- open reduction if closed reduction unsuccessful

SURGICAL ANATOMY

- mechanism of injury is a pull on the hand with the forearm in pronation
- radial head is pulled distal to the annular ligament, which usually remains intact

APPROACHES

Manipulation Technique

- anesthesia usually is not required.
- reduce by supinating the forearm fully, with the elbow flexed at approximately 90°

POSTOPERATIVE MANAGEMENT

- sling only for comfort

REHABILITATION

- in younger child (6 months to 3 years), normal activity begins in minutes
- in older child (>3 years), some pain may limit activity for a few days because of possible partial tears of the annular ligament

COMPLICATIONS

- none other than occasional recurrence

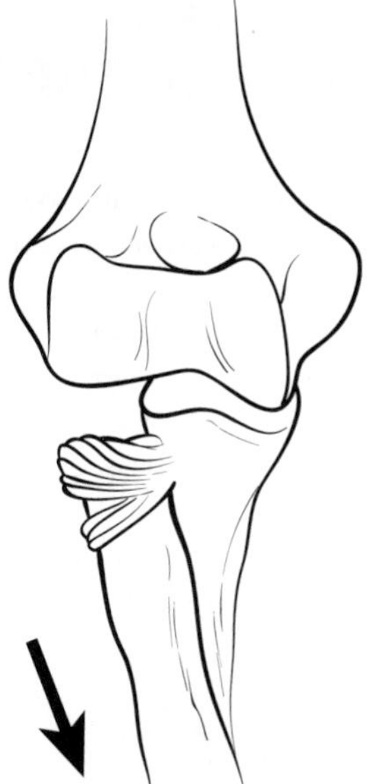

SELECTED REFERENCES

Choung W, Heinrich SD. Acute annular ligament interposition into the radiocapitellar joint in children (nurse maid's elbow). J Pediatr Orthop 1995;15:454.

Salter RB, Zaltz C. Anatomic investigations of the mechanism of injury and pathologic anatomy of "pulled elbow" in young children. Clin Orthop 1971;77:141.

NOTES

ELBOW

CLOSED TREATMENT OF RADIAL HEAD FRACTURE

CPT code	**24650 closed treatment of radial head or neck fracture, without manipulation**
	24655 closed treatment of radial head or neck fracture, with manipulation
ICD-9 codes	**813.05 closed radial head fracture**
	813.06 closed radial neck fracture
	813.15 open radial head fracture
	813.16 open radial neck fracture

Mason classification

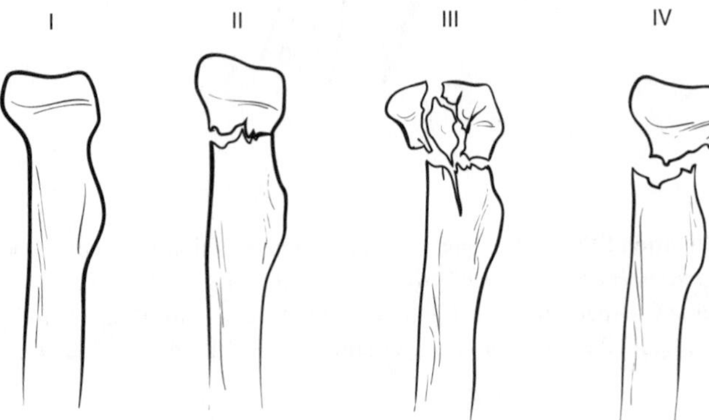

INDICATIONS

- nondisplaced type I radial head or neck fractures (in situ)
- most commonly for a displaced radial neck fracture in a skeletally immature patient

ALTERNATIVE TREATMENTS

- closed reduction with percutaneous pin fixation
- open reduction with internal fixation
- partial excision of radial head fragment

POSTOPERATIVE MANAGEMENT

- brief initial immobilization in long arm splint including the wrist
- limit initial immobilization to less than 3 weeks to limit stiffness

REHABILITATION

- protected active range of motion during fracture healing (first 4–6 weeks)
- progress to full mobility when clinically nontender and fracture is stable

COMPLICATIONS

- elbow flexion contracture, often mild, sometimes occurs despite early aggressive active range of motion
- stiffness secondary to prolonged immobilization
- limited motion secondary to unrecognized osteochondral fragments or fracture displacement

SELECTED REFERENCES

Caputo AE, Mazzocca AD. Radial head fractures. Tech Orthop 2000;15:128–137.

Morrey BF. Current concepts in the treatment of fractures of the radial head, the olecranon, and the coronoid. Instr Course Lect 1995;44:175–185.

NOTES

OPEN TREATMENT OF RADIAL HEAD FRACTURE

CPT code **24665 open treatment of radial head or neck fracture, with or without internal fixation or radial head excision**

ICD-9 code **813.05 radial head fracture**

INDICATIONS

- stable fractures without mechanical block to forearm rotation can be treated with early motion
- open reduction for "fixable" fragments with articular step-off

ALTERNATIVE TREATMENT(S)

- early motion, with or without delayed excision
- early excision and replacement

SURGICAL ANATOMY (see p. 70, 24130)

Incision

- starts 2–3 cm proximal to the lateral epicondyle and curves dorsal to it to extend parallel to the radius for 3–4 cm

APPROACH

Surgical Technique

Direct reduction by using a dental pick with provisional fixation with 1.0-mm K-wire followed by definitive stabilization (2.0-mm screws, miniplates) that should be placed so as to not limit rotation. Focus should be on reestablishing normal ligamentous and capsular relations.

POSTOPERATIVE MANAGEMENT

- well-padded splint with elevation to avoid edema

REHABILITATION

- start range of motion as soon as possible after surgery
- use removable posterior splint for 3–4 weeks
- closed treatment with early motion
- radial head replacement for irreparable fractures with instability
- radial head excision for irreparable fractures without ligamentous laxity

COMPLICATIONS

- joint stiffness
- non-union
- hardware failure

SELECTED REFERENCES

King GJ, Evans DC, Kellam JF. Open reduction internal fixation of radial head fractures. J Orthop Trauma 1991;5:21–28.

Teasdall R, Savoie FH, Hughes JL. Comminuted fractures of the proximal radius and ulna. Clin Orthop 1993;2920:37–47.

NOTES

CLOSED TREATMENT OF OLECRANON FRACTURE

CPT code **24670 closed treatment of ulnar fracture, proximal end (olecranon process); without manipulation**

ICD-9 codes **813.01 closed olecranon fracture**
813.04 other or unspecified closed fractures of the proximal end of the ulna

INDICATIONS

- nondisplaced or minimally displaced fractures of the olecranon without any ulnohumeral instability
- active extension demonstrable

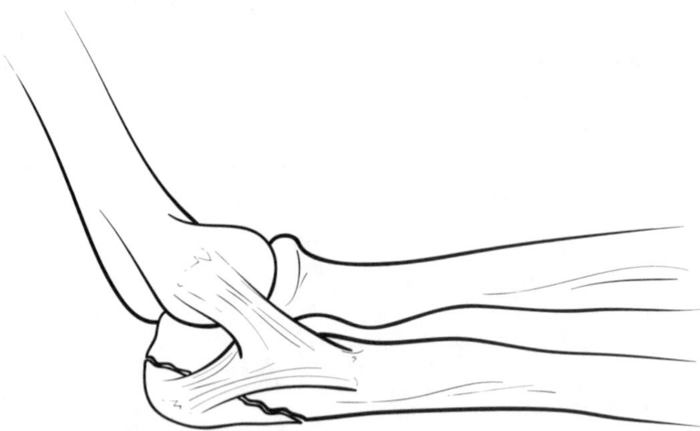

ALTERNATIVE TREATMENT

- with significant displacement, joint step-off, or any ulnohumeral instability, open reduction–internal fixation should be considered

POSTOPERATIVE MANAGEMENT

- brief immobilization in long arm splint with elbow flexed to 45–90°

REHABILITATION

- immobilize for 2–3 weeks and then begin active motion or begin protected active motion sooner

COMPLICATIONS

- displacement with early motion; rare, if nondisplaced
- stiffness with prolonged immobilization (>3 weeks)

SELECTED REFERENCES

Colton CL. Fractures of the olecranon in adults: classification and management. Injury 1980;5:121.

Morrey BF. Current concepts in the treatment of fractures of the radial head, the olecranon, and the coronoid. J Bone Joint Surg 1995;77A:316–127.

NOTES

OPEN TREATMENT OF OLECRANON FRACTURE

CPT code **24685 open treatment of ulnar fracture proximal end (olecranon process), with or without internal or external fixation**

ICD-9 codes
813.01 closed olecranon fracture
813.04 other or unspecified closed fractures of the proximal end of the ulna
813.11 open olecranon fracture
813.14 other or unspecified open fractures of the proximal end of the ulna

INDICATIONS

- displaced olecranon fractures
- any evidence of elbow joint subluxation or dislocation

ALTERNATIVE TREATMENTS

- excision of proximal olecranon fragment and reattachment of triceps tendon (less than 50% articular involvement)
- closed treatment with cast or splint immobilization in extension (not appropriate with joint subluxation or dislocation)
- fixation options
    - tension band wire (K-wire and wire spool)
    - intramedullary screw fixation, with or without tension band
    - bicortical screw fixation
    - plate fixation; consider a rigid plate (i.e., 3.5 low contact dynamic compression plate [LCDCP]) for comminution or coronoid involvement or joint subluxation

SURGICAL ANATOMY

Incision

- skin incision, slightly lateral to avoid scar tenderness

APPROACH

- direct posterior

Surgical Techniques

- supine position with the arm over the chest or lateral decubitus with the upper arm over the arm holder (preferred because the long head of the triceps is relaxed)
- fracture site exposure and joint debridement

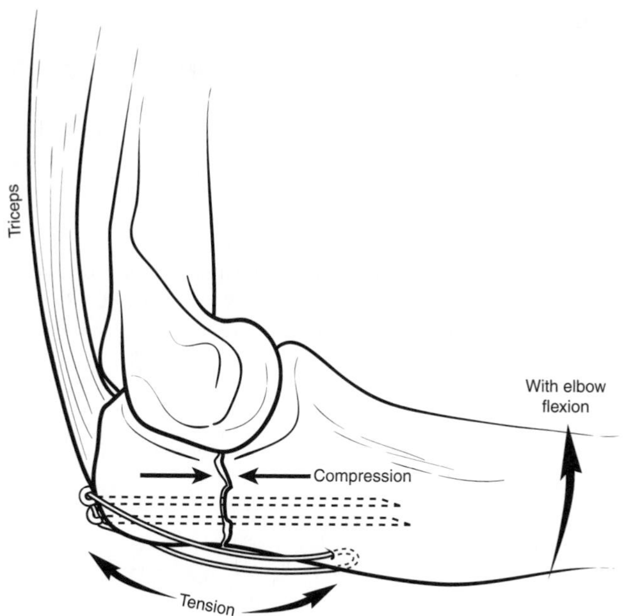

- for K-wire or tension band, place K-wire or band retrograde in the proximal fragment, reduce the fracture, and then antegrade to engage the anterior cortex (important to minimize wire backing out) (not illustrated)
- transverse drill hole in ulna cortex distally to pass spool wire
- medial and lateral tightening of wire for even compression (not illustrated)
- bend end of K-wires and spool wire away from subcutaneous areas of the proximal ulna
- layer closure

POSTOPERATIVE MANAGEMENT

- consider posterior splint for comfort

REHABILITATION

- with stable fixation, begin gravity-assisted extension within 2 weeks
- active assisted motion, non-weight-bearing until fracture has healed (usually about 6 weeks)

COMPLICATIONS

- hardware prominence or backout and subcutaneous irritation, often requiring removal
- non-union from inadequate fixation for fracture involvement distal to and/or involving the coronoid process

SELECTED REFERENCES

Morrey BF. Current concepts in the treatment of fractures of the radial head, the olecranon, and the coronoid. Instruct Course Lect 1995;44:175–185.

Wolfgang G, Burke F, Bush D, et al. Surgical treatment of displaced olecranon fractures by tension band wiring technique. Clin Orthop 1987;224:192.

NOTES

P A R T I V

FOREARM & WRIST

RELEASE DEQUERVAIN'S TENOSYNOVITIS

CPT code **25000 incision, extensor tendon sheath, wrist (e.g., deQuervain's disease)**

ICD-9 code **727.04 deQuervain's disease**

INDICATIONS

- failure of conservative management including nonsteroidal anti-inflammatory drugs, steroid injection, therapy, splinting

ALTERNATIVE TREATMENT

- conservative management as above

SURGICAL ANATOMY

Incision
- dorsalradial 0.5 cm proximal to radial styloid

APPROACHES

Surgical Techniques
- protect radial sensory branches
- open first dorsal extensor compartment (abductor pollicis longus and extensor pollicis brevis)
- search for separate EPB compartments

POSTOPERATIVE MANAGEMENT

- immediate thumb gutter splint and mobilize to tolerance

REHABILITATION

- usually not necessary

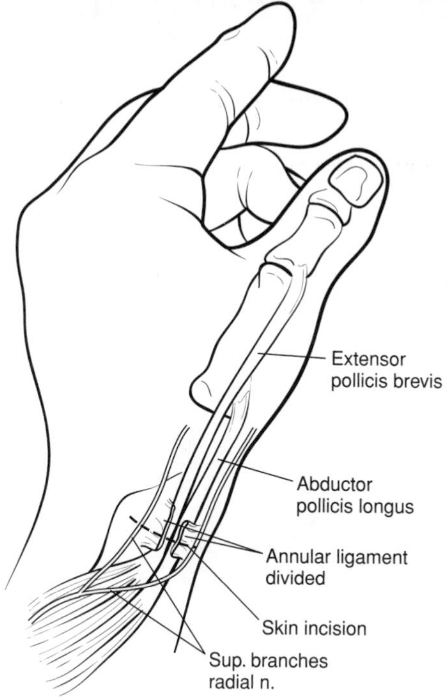

COMPLICATIONS

- iatrogenic injury to the superficial branch of the radial sensory nerve
- volar subluxation of tendons

SELECTED REFERENCES

Ta K, Thomson JG. Patient satisfaction and outcomes for deQuervain's tenosynovitis. J Hand Surg 1999;24A;1071–1077.

Witt J, Gelberman RH. Treatment of deQuervain's tenosynovitis. J Bone Joint Surg 1991;73A:219–221.

EXCISION OF WRIST GANGLION

CPT code **25111 excision of ganglion, wrist (dorsal or volar); primary**

ICD-9 code **727.41 ganglion of the joint**

INDICATIONS

- dysfunction, pain, or cosmetic abnormality despite observation, nonsteroidal anti-inflammatory drugs, recurrence after aspiration

ALTERNATIVE TREATMENTS

- aspiration
- treat only if symptomatic

SURGICAL ANATOMY

Incision
- dorsal
- volar

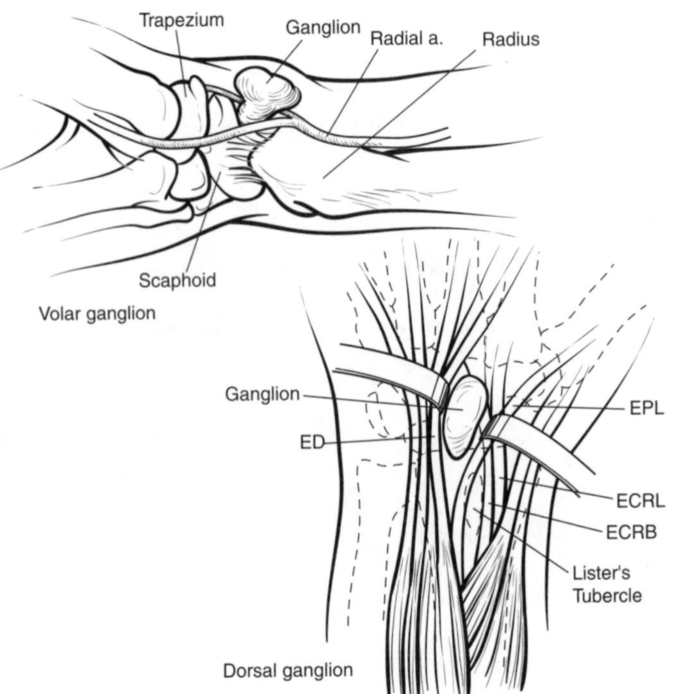

APPROACHES

Surgical Techniques

- position supine or upper extremity (UE) on arm table or in tourniquet
- transverse incision (dorsal), longitudinal, or transverse incision (volar)
- identify and protect extensor and flexor tendons, radial artery (volar), and dorsal sensory nerves
- dissect ganglion from surrounding tissue and excise portion of wrist capsule at site of cyst
- excise stalk to intercarpal joint (dorsal to scapholunate joint and volar to scaphoradial or scaphotrapezial joint are most common) and preserve intercarpal ligament
- closure

POSTOPERATIVE MANAGEMENT

- dressing and splint for 7–10 days
- instruct in early digital motion
- suture removal after 7–10 days

REHABILITATION

- active and passive range of motion exercises for hand and wrist
- strengthening program

COMPLICATIONS

- infection
- recurrence
- nerve, tendon, and vessel injuries
- pain and stiffness
- complex regional pain syndrome (reflex sympathetic dystrophy)
- wrist instability (if intercarpal ligaments injured)

SELECTED REFERENCES

Green DP, Hotchkiss RN, Pederson WC, eds. Green's operative hand surgery. New York: Churchill Livingstone, 1999.

Gelberman RH, ed. Master techniques in orthopaedic surgery: the wrist. New York: Raven Press, 1994.

NOTES

CLOSED TREATMENT OF RADIAL SHAFT FRACTURE

CPT code **25500 closed treatment of radial shaft fracture; without manipulation**

ICD-9 code **813.21 fracture of radial shaft**

INDICATIONS

- nondisplaced fracture of the radial shaft
- can accept ≤10° angulation without subluxation of the proximal or distal radioulnar joints

ALTERNATIVE TREATMENTS

- long arm cast
- fracture brace
- open reduction-internal fixation

SURGICAL ANATOMY

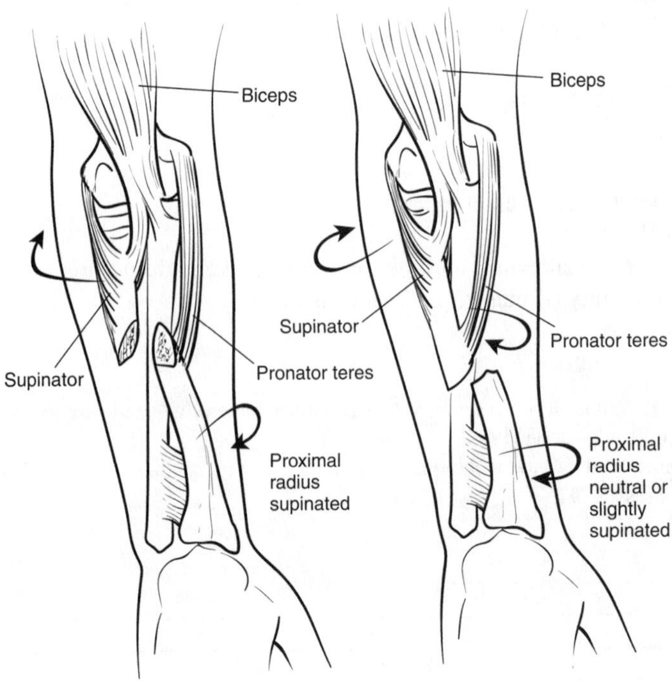

- anatomic position of fracture should determine position of forearm rotation for long arm cast

Cast Position
- immobilize forearm in maximum supination for fractures distal to the biceps and supinator insertion and proximal to pronator teres insertion
- immobilize forearm in neutral to slight supination for fractures distal to pronator teres insertion

POSTOPERATIVE MANAGEMENT

- remove long arm cast or brace at 6 weeks
- early digital and shoulder motion during immobilization period

REHABILITATION

- active and passive range of motion program beginning at 6 weeks
- strengthening program

COMPLICATIONS

- fracture displacement (requires close clinical and radiographic follow-up)
- non-union, delayed union, and malunion
- neurovascular compromise and compartment syndrome (high index of suspicion)
- skin compromise from cast
- complex regional pain syndrome (reflex sympathetic dystrophy)
- pain and stiffness

SELECTED REFERENCE

Rockwood CA, Green DP, Heckman JD, et al, eds. Rockwood and Green's fractures in adults. Philadelphia: Lippincott-Williams & Wilkins, 2001.

NOTES

OPEN TREATMENT OF RADIAL SHAFT FRACTURE

CPT code **25525** **open treatment of radial shaft fracture, with internal and/or external fixation and closed treatment of dislocation of distal radioulnar joint (Galeazzi fracture and dislocation), with or without percutaneous skeletal fixation**

ICD-9 codes **813.21** **fracture radial shaft**
833.01 **closed dislocation radioulnar joint**

INDICATIONS

- displaced fractures in adults; failure of closed reduction in children <10 years
- open fracture(s)
- setting of multiple trauma
- arterial compromise

APPROACHES

Surgical Techniques

- supine position or upper extremity on arm board or in tourniquet
- longitudinal incision
- incise fascia
- FCR/BR interval (volar); ECRB/EDC interval (dorsal)
- protect radial artery and elevate pronator teres, FPL, and pronator quadratus (volar)
- identify supinator, dissect and protect posterior interosseous nerve (PIN), and elevate supinator (dorsal)
- reduce fracture and apply plate (3.5 low contact dynamic compression plate [LCDCP] with 3 screws both proximal and distal to fracture site)
- closure
- if distal radioulnar joint (DRUJ) stable postreduction; use long arm splint with forearm in supination; if unstable, reduce and pin with 1 or 2 K-wires

FIXATION OPTIONS

- plate and screws (most common)
- intramedullary flexible rodding
- external fixation
- K-wires (for unstable DRUJ)

SURGICAL ANATOMY

Incision

- dorsal: Thompson (most commonly used for fractures of the proximal-half radius)

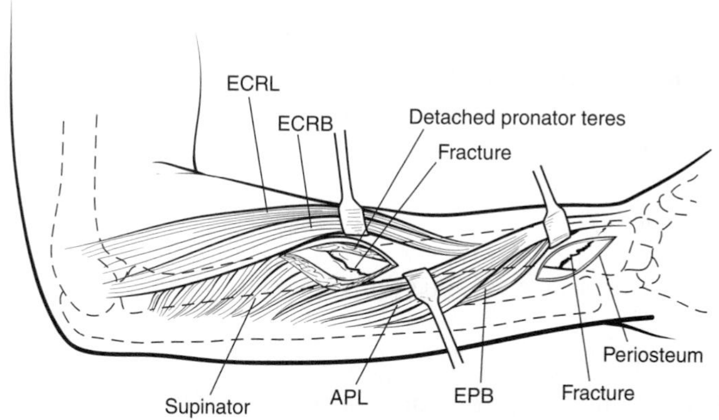

- volar: Henry (most commonly used for fractures of the distal-half radius)

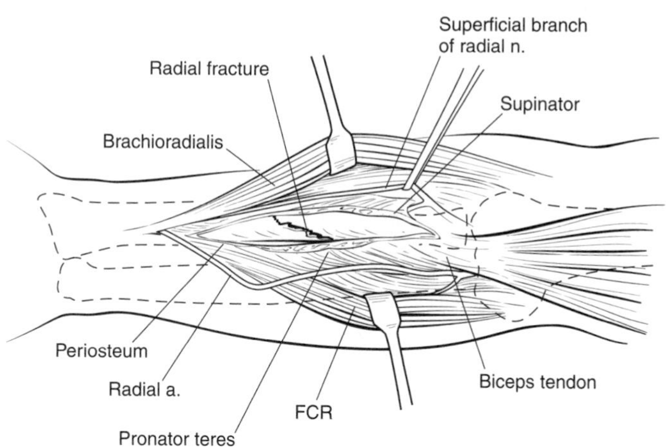

POSTOPERATIVE MANAGEMENT

- remove sutures after 7–10 days
- long arm cast for 6 weeks (elbow at 90º flexion; forearm in full supination)
- with DRUJ fixation, remove K-wire(s) at 4–6 weeks

REHABILITATION

- active and passive range of motion program
- strengthening program

COMPLICATIONS

- infection
- nerve and vessel injuries (PIN); compartment syndrome
- delayed union, non-union, or malunion
- forearm synostosis
- pain and stiffness
- DRUJ instability
- RSD
- refracture after plate removal (generally, do not)

SELECTED REFERENCES

Jupiter JB, Kellam JF. Diaphyseal fractures of the forearm. In: Browner BD et al, eds. Skeletal trauma, 2/e. Philadelphia: WB Saunders, 1998.

Rockwood CA, Green DP, Heckman JD, et al, eds. Rockwood and Green's fractures in adults. Philadelphia: Lippincott, Williams & Wilkins, 2001.

Wiss DA. Master techniques in orthopaedic surgery. In: Fractures. Philadelphia: Lippincott-Raven, 1998.

NOTES

CLOSED TREATMENT OF ULNAR SHAFT FRACTURE

CPT code **25530 closed treatment of ulnar shaft fracture; without manipulation**

ICD-9 code **813.22 closed fracture of ulnar shaft**

INDICATIONS

- fractures of the ulnar shaft where length is maintained and interosseous ligament is not shortened
- treatment goal is the preservation of supination and pronation

ALTERNATIVE TREATMENT(S)

- open reduction–internal fixation
- intramedullary nailing

SURGICAL ANATOMY

Management

- midshaft ulna is subcutaneous
- limited muscle coverage correlated with presumed lower vascularity and slower healing
- long arm cast in supination until early callus seen (3–4 weeks), then short arm cast with interosseous mold (3–4 weeks)

REHABILITATION

- elbow range of motion when short arm cast applied
- postoperative emphasis is on supination and pronation

COMPLICATIONS

- displacement
- loss of pronation and supination (accept ≤10° angulation of midshaft fracture)

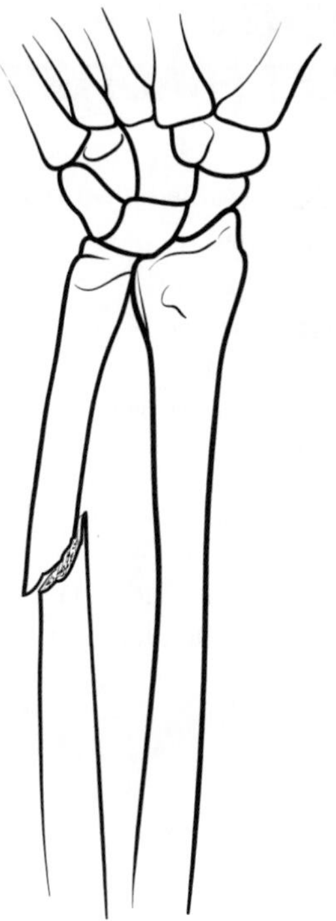

FOREARM & WRIST

NOTES

OPEN TREATMENT OF ULNAR SHAFT FRACTURE

CPT code	**25545**	**open treatment of ulnar shaft fracture; with or without internal or external fixation**
ICD-9 codes	**813.03**	**Monteggia's fracture**
	813.2	**shaft, closed**
	813	**fracture of radius and ulna**
	813.3	**shaft, open**

INDICATIONS

- combined fractures of the radius and ulna
- displaced isolated fracture of the ulna
- Monteggia fracture
- open fracture

ALTERNATIVE TREATMENTS

- closed treatment
- intramedullary nailing
- open reduction–internal fixation (most common)
- external fixation

SURGICAL ANATOMY

Incision

- incision runs parallel to the ulnar crest

APPROACHES

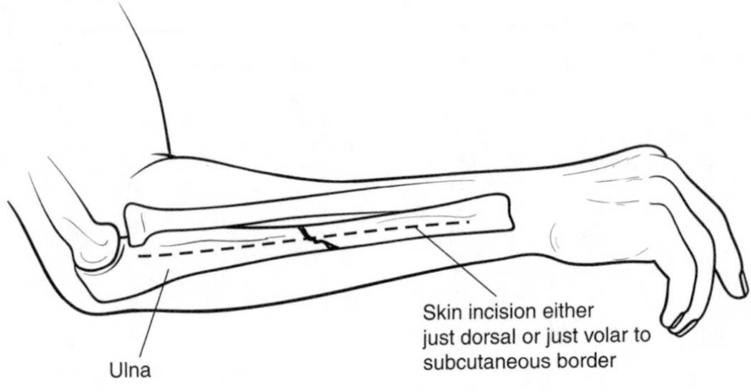

Surgical Techniques

- patient supine
- use of tourniquet is case dependent
- prep out iliac crest as needed (bone graft >50% displacement or comminution)
- place 3.5 low contact dynamic compression plate dorsally

POSTOPERATIVE MANAGEMENT

- functional after treatment with soft splint in reliable patients
- early range of motion started after 24–48 hours of elevation

REHABILITATION

- elbow range of motion
- postoperative emphasis on supination and pronation

COMPLICATIONS

- non-union and malunion
- synostosis (avoid interosseous dissection or retractors)
- loss of pronation and supination
- refracture after implant removal (generally not recommended)

SELECTED REFERENCES

Chapman MW, Gordon JE, Zissimos AG. Compression-plate fixation of acute fractures of the diaphyses of the radius and ulna. J Bone Joint Surg 1989;71:159–169.

Hertel R, Pisan M, Lambert S, et al. Plate osteosynthesis of diaphyseal fractures of the radius and ulna. Injury 1996;27:545–548.

NOTES

CLOSED TREATMENT OF RADIAL AND ULNAR FRACTURES

CPT code **25560 closed treatment of radial and ulnar shaft fractures; without manipulation**

ICD-9 code **813 fracture of radius and ulna**

INDICATIONS

- low-energy fractures with minimal comminution
- angulation <10° in mid-diaphysis; can accept up to 30° in the sagittal plane in the distal metaphysis
- isolated radius or ulna (nightstick)-type fractures are more amenable to closed treatment
- both bone fractures in children ≤10 years generally should be treated closed; maintenance of rotation alignment is important

ALTERNATIVE TREATMENTS

- open reduction–internal fixation
- intramedullary rodding

MANAGEMENT

- both bone and isolated ulnar fractures require a long arm cast to prevent rotational deformity
- employ interosseous mold to control fracture hydrostatically
- in adult, change to short arm cast in 4 weeks
- typically requires 6–8 weeks of immobilization for healing

REHABILITATION

- active range of motion elbow once short arm cast is applied
- focus on pronation and supination: have patient hold a ruler in the hand and make it parallel to the floor

COMPLICATIONS

- limited range of motion, particularly when the mid-diaphyseal angulation is >10°
- synosthosis is rare without surgical intervention
- undiagnosed additional elbow or wrist pathology: rule out Galeazzi or Montaggia equivalents

NOTES

CLOSED TREATMENT OF DISTAL RADIUS FRACTURE

CPT code **25600 closed treatment of distal radial (e.g., Colles or Smith type) or epiphyseal separation, with or without fracture of ulnar styloid; without manipulation**

ICD-9 codes **813.41 Colles' fracture; Smith's fracture** **(see diagram p. 113)**
813.42 other fractures of distal end of radius (alone)

INDICATIONS

Distal radius fractures that are nondisplaced or minimally displaced which can be manipulated into acceptable alignment, or where the patient physiologically cannot tolerate operative intervention

ALTERNATIVE TREATMENTS

- percutaneous external fixation
- percutaneous pinning of the distal radius for potentially unstable fractures
- open reduction–internal fixation

APPROACHES

- closed reduction of the distal radius as necessary under hematoma block and intravenous sedation; finger traps and countertraction are helpful
- reduction manuever to correct dorsal angulation, radial shortening, or loss of radial inclination
- well-padded sugar-tong splint; elbow is held in neutral rotation; wrist in slight (not severe) flexion and ulnar deviation; finger metacarpal phalangeal (MCP) and interphalangeal (IP) joints should be free for motion
- radiographs (posteroanterior, lateral and oblique) in plaster to confirm reduction
- recheck median nerve after reduction maneuver

POSTINJURY MANAGEMENT

- elevation of extremity
- regular radiographic evaluation (every 7–10 days) for 2–4 weeks
- active and passive finger range of motion
- snug-fitting splint or cast; change when necessary

REHABILITATION

- active range of wrist motion when fracture is healed (usually begun at approximately 6 weeks)
- strengthening; return to normal activities 6–10 weeks after fracture

COMPLICATIONS

- finger swelling, stiffness
- wrist stiffness
- instability and pain distal radial ulnar joint (DRUJ)
- median nerve compression (early or late)
- complex regional pain syndrome (reflex sympathetic dystrophy)
- malunion

SELECTED REFERENCES

Frykman G. Fracture of the distal radius including sequelae—shoulder-hand-finger syndrome, disturbance in the distal radioulnar joint and impairment of nerve function. Acta Orthop Scand 1967;108(suppl):1–153.

Newport ML. Colles' fracture: managing a common upper extremity injury. J Musculoskel Med 2000;17:292–301.

NOTES

OPEN TREATMENT OF DISTAL RADIUS FRACTURE

CPT code **25620 open treatment of distal radial fracture (e.g., Colles or Smith type) or epiphyseal separation, with or without fracture of ulnar styloid, with or without internal or external fixation**

ICD-9 code **813.41 Colles' fracture; Smith's fracture**

INDICATIONS

- distal radius angulation (>15° dorsal or volar), significant shortening, intra-articular step-off >2 mm, incongruity of DRUJ

ALTERNATIVE TREATMENTS

- closed reduction and casting
- percutaneous pinning and casting
- external fixation with or without percutaneous pinning

SURGICAL ANATOMY

Incisions
- dorsal
- volar

APPROACHES

Surgical Techniques
- supine
- arm table
- tourniquet upper extremity
- dorsal
  - incision over fourth dorsal compartment
  - protect dorsal sensory nerves
  - open fourth compartment, EDC reflected ulnarly
  - open third compartment, EPL reflected radially
  - longitudinal periosteal and capsular (as necessary) incision
  - provisional K-wire fixation, as necessary
  - minifluoroscopic confirmation of reduction
  - final fixation with plates, screws, or K-wires, as selected
  - bone grafting, as necessary (with significant comminution)
  - repair capsule and dorsal retinaculum
  - bulky dressing with plaster splint

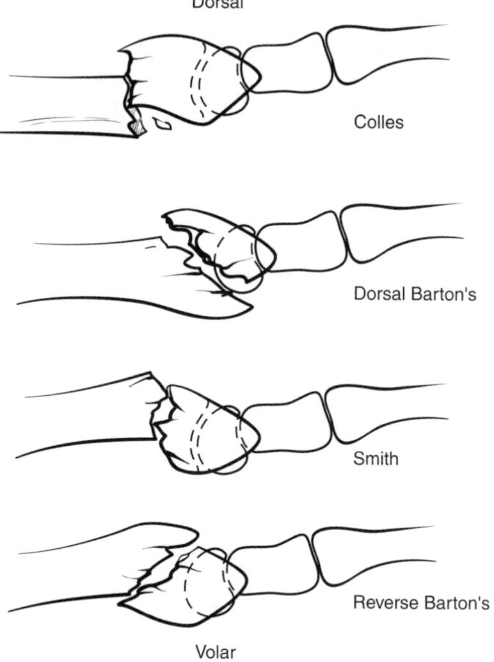

- volar
  - incision (longitudinal) just radial to FCR
  - FCR reflected ulnarly, radial artery reflected radially
  - pronator quadratus incised off radial aspect radius, reflected ulnarly
  - volar capsule and ligaments are not violated
  - provisional fixation, as necessary
  - minifluoroscopic confirmation reduction
  - final fixation with plate, screws, or K-wires

POSTOPERATIVE MANAGEMENT

- elevation
- careful attention to active finger range of motion
- mobilization dependent on strength and stability of construct

REHABILITATION

- immediate active and passive finger range of motion
- active wrist range of motion when construct is stable, usually before 6 weeks
- begin strengthening; return to normal activities at 6–10 weeks

COMPLICATIONS

- swelling and stiffness in fingers
- lost wrist range of motion
- complex regional pain syndrome (reflex sympathetic dystrophy)
- median nerve compression (early or late)
- infection (soft tissue and osteomyelitis)
- malunion

NOTES

P A R T V

HAND

CLOSED TREATMENT OF SCAPHOID FRACTURE

CPT code **25622 closed treatment of carpal scaphoid (navicular) fracture, without manipulation**

ICD-9 code **814.01 closed fracture of navicular (scaphoid) bone of wrist**

INDICATION

- nondisplaced fracture of scaphoid or fracture displaced <1 mm

ALTERNATIVE TREATMENTS

- percutaneous internal fixation through a dorsal or volar approach may decrease the length of treatment and extent of immobilization

SUGGESTED TREATMENT

- any nondisplaced fracture of scaphoid or suspected fracture should be treated initially in the emergency department with a long arm thumb spica splint or cast, depending on initial swelling
- the wrist is placed in slight flexion and radial deviation, with the thumb in opposition.
- the elbow is placed in 90° flexion and neutral supination and pronation.
- long-term management depends on the location of the fracture
- distal tubercle fractures heal readily within 6 weeks and probably do not require long arm casting.
- mid-waist fractures, if of a stable configuration (transverse or horizontal oblique), require longer immobilization, usually 6–10 weeks of immobilization, half in a long arm thumb spica and half in a short arm thumb spica.
- mid-waist fractures of an unstable configuration (vertical oblique) probably should be managed in a long arm thumb spica for longer (6–8 weeks) and then changed to a short arm thumb spica until fracture healing (average total immobilization of 10–16 weeks).
- proximal pole fractures can take 16–20 weeks to heal, usually with 6 weeks in a long arm cast and the remainder in a short arm thumb spica cast.

POSTINJURY MANAGEMENT

- After radiographs and clinical examination appear to show healing, some recommend computed tomography to confirm fracture repair.

REHABILITATION

- Wrist stiffness is a common consequence of long-term immobilizaton and most patients will benefit from occupational therapy to mobilize and strengthen the wrist and hand.

COMPLICATIONS

- stiffness and pain ("postscaphoid syndrome").
- non-union: The scaphoid bone is almost entirely intracapsular and the fracture is continuously bathed in joint fluid, which can increase the rate of non-union formation.
- the fracture pattern also may contribute to instability and micromotion.
- the position of the fracture also contributes to the rate of non-union, with proximal pole fractures having a significantly higher rate of non-union than mid-waist fractures.
- the blood supply to the scaphoid relies on two vessels that enter the distal pole and supply the entire length of the bone. Fractures of the waist and especially the proximal pole are subject to avascular necrosis, which also contributes to non-union formation.

SELECTED REFERENCES

Gelberman RH, Menon J. The vascularity of the scaphoid bone. J Hand Surg 1980; 5:508–513.

Gellman H, Caputo RJ, Carter V, et al. Comparison of short and long thumb-spica casts for non-displaced fractures of the carpal scaphoid. J Bone Joint Surg 1989; 71A:354–357.

NOTES

CLOSED TREATMENT OF CARPAL FRACTURE

CPT code 25630 closed treatment of carpal bone fracture (excluding carpal scaphoid-navicular), without manipulation, each bone

ICD-9 codes
- 814.07 capitate
- 814.08 hamate
- 814.02 lunate
- 814.04 pisiform
- 814.06 trapezoid
- 814.05 trapezium

INDICATIONS

- nondisplaced fractures of the lunate, triquetrum, hamate, capitate, trapezoid, or trapezium

ALTERNATIVE TREATMENT

- percutaneous pinning, if multiple fractures

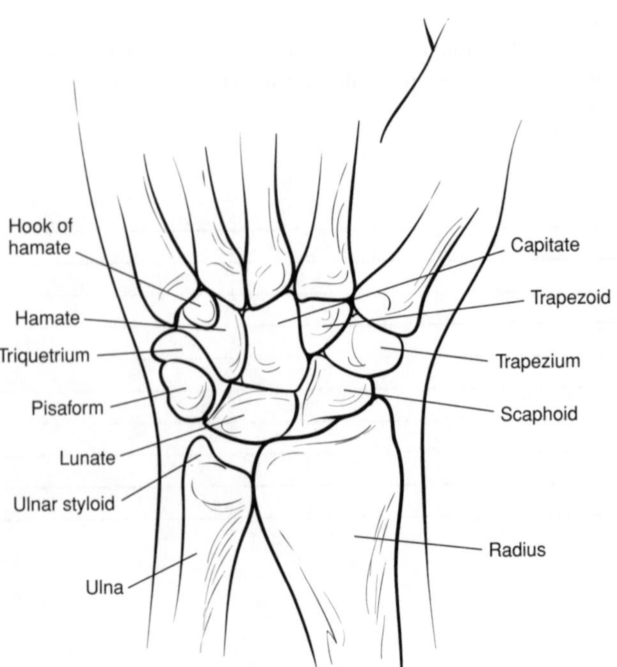

DIAGNOSIS

- high index of suspicion required; special views may be required
- pisiform: supination oblique, carpal tunnel view
- trapezium: Bett's view, carpal tunnel view
- hamate hook: supination oblique (with dorsiflexion), carpal tunnel view

MANAGEMENT

- short arm casting for 4–6 weeks; include thumb and index for trapezial and trapezoid fractures

REHABILITATION

- active range of motion exercises after fracture is healed (6 weeks)

COMPLICATIONS

- missed carpal instability
- avascular necrosis (AVN) (lunate, capitate, pisiform)
- non-union (lunate, hook of hamate, pisiform)

SELECTED REFERENCE

Amadio PC, Taleisnik J. Fractures of the carpal bones. In: Green DP, ed. Operative hand surgery, 3rd ed. New York: Churchill Livingtone, 1999:799–860.

NOTES

CLOSED TREATMENT OF LUNATE DISLOCATION

CPT code **25690 closed treatment of lunate dislocation, with manipulation**

ICD-9 code **833.00 closed dislocation of wrist**

INDICATION

- acute dislocations

ALTERNATIVE TREATMENTS

Surgical Anatomy

- volar lunate dislocation: lunate fossa is empty, lunate is volar, and remainder of carpus is colinear with the radius
- dorsal lunate dislocation (rare): lunate fossa is empty, lunate is dorsal, and remainder of carpus in nearly colinear with the longitudinal axis of the radius

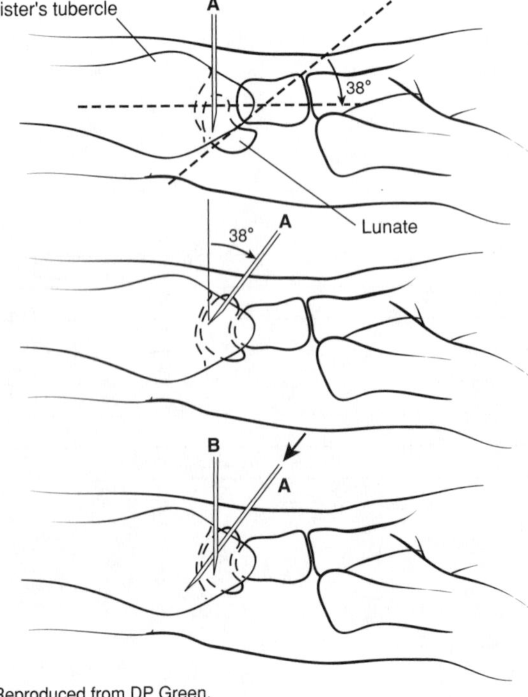

Reproduced from DP Green.

APPROACHES

Manipulation Technique for Volar Lunate Dislocation

- longitudinal manual traction
- carpus is extended and then flexed, maintaining volar pressure on the lunate
- hematoma block with 1% Lidocaine plain combined with 0.25% Marcaine
- this may need to be combined with 3 point pressure thumb volar to achieve best results
- pad the extremity well and place sugar tong splint in intrinsic–plus position
- obtain postreduction x-ray

POSTOPERATIVE MANAGEMENT

- wrist is splinted in neutral position
- posteroanterior and lateral postreduction x-rays are obtained
- cast once edema reduced
- requires ORIF if not anatomic

COMPLICATIONS

- inadequate reduction
- persistent carpal tunnel syndrome
- high incidence of chronic instability

SELECTED REFERENCES

Green DP, Hotchkiss RN, Pederson WC, eds. Green's operative hand surgery. New York: Churchill Livingston, 1999.

Hertzberg G, Comtet JJ, Linscheid RL, et al. Perilunate dislocations and fracture-dislocations: a multicenter study. J Hand Surg Am 1993;18(5):768–779.

Lavernia CJ, Cohen MS, Taleisnik J. Treatment of scapholunate dissociation by ligamentous repair and capsulodesis. J Hand Surg Am 1992;17:354.

NOTES

TRIGGER FINGER RELEASE

CPT code **26055 tendon sheath incision (e.g., for trigger finger)**

ICD-9 code **727.03 trigger finger (acquired)**

INDICATIONS

- failure of conservative therapy including splinting, rest, nonsteroidal anti-inflammatory drugs, and steroid injection (avoid tendon)
- frequent or persistent locking

ALTERNATIVE TREATMENT

- percutaneous trigger finger release

SURGICAL ANATOMY

Incision

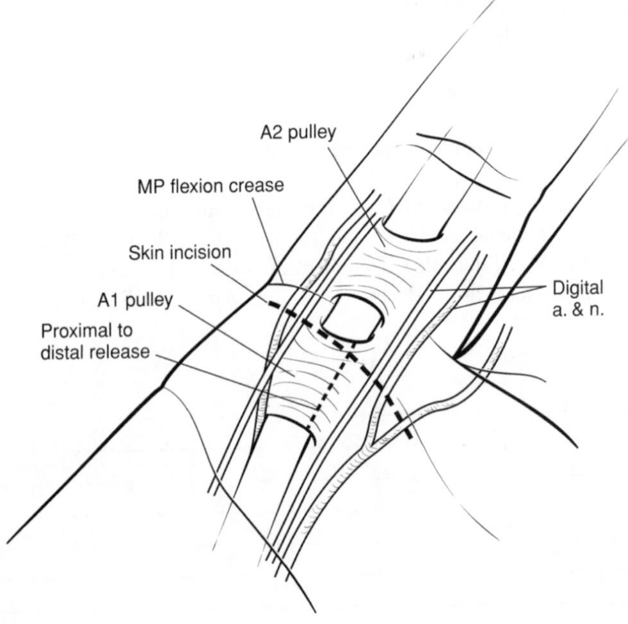

APPROACHES

- oblique skin incision over distal palmar crease provides access to proximal (A1) annular pulley

Surgical Technique

- neurovascular bundles are retracted
- A-1 pulley is incised from proximal to distal along side of pulley
- 3-mm portion of pulley is resected
- palmar fascia overlying pulley is also incised

POSTOPERATIVE MANAGEMENT

- bulky hand dressing for 2 days

REHABILITATION

- active range of motion

COMPLICATIONS

- digital nerve injury
- bowstringing secondary to inadvertant A-2 pulley release
- inadequate release

NOTES

EXTENSOR TENDON REPAIR, FINGER

CPT code **26418 repair extensor tendon, finger, primary or secondary; without free graft, each tendon**

ICD-9 code **727.63 extensor tendon rupture of the hand and wrist**

ALTERNATIVE TREATMENTS

- acute closed zone I and II injuries are indications for nonsurgical treatment (splint)
- chronic extensor tendon deficit is reconstructed by tendon transfer

SURGICAL ANATOMY

- the extensor tendons, from the radial side to the ulnar side of the wrist, are EPB, EPL, EIP, EDC, and EDM
- level of extensor tendon injury is divided into nine zones from the distal interphalengeal (DIP) joint to the proximal forearm

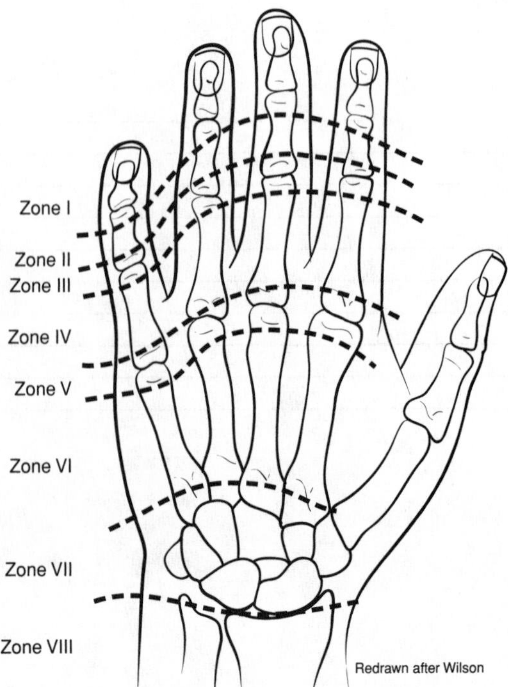

APPROACHES

Surgical Techniques

- index–little fingers
  - suture technique: Kleinert modification of Bunnell's technique
  - important not to shorten excessively to prevent the restriction of metacarpal phalangeal (MCP) and proximal interphalengeal (PIP) flexion
  - nonresorbable 4-0 or 5-0 suture (3-0 is best at zone VIII)

• zone I:	(chronic mallet)	terminal tendon advancement
	(chronic mallet with swan neck)	superficial tenodesis, or spiral oblique retinacular ligament (SORL) reconstruction
• zone II:	(open)	same as for zone I—anatomic repair
• zone III:	(open acute)	repair of the central slip supplemented with transarticular K-wire for at least 6 weeks
	(chronic flexible Boutonniere)	anatomic reconstruction of the central slip
	(chronic rigid Boutonniere)	splint to remove contracture and anatomic reconstruction of the central slip
• zone IV:		repair
• zone V:	(human bite)	usually a partial—do not repair; debride and use antibiotics
	(sagittal band)	debride, repair and reinforcement
• zone VI:		repair
• zone VII:		repair with retinacular excision or transposition
• zone VIII:		central core suture

- Thumb

• zones I and II:		repair similar to that of digits
• zone III:		repair EPL and EPB
• zones IV and V:	(acute)	3-0 or 4-0 nonabsorbable suture
	(old or closed)	EIP to EPL tendon transfer, intercalated tendon graft

COMPLICATIONS

- loss of active flexion if too tight imbrication or shortening

SELECTED REFERENCES

Newport ML. Extensor tendon injuries in the hand. J Am Acad Orthop Surg 1997;5(2):59–66.

CLOSED TREATMENT OF MALLET FINGER

CPT code **26432 closed treatment of distal extensor tendon insertion, with or without percutaneous pinning**

ICD-9 code **736.1 mallet finger**

INDICATION

- standard treatment for extensor mechanism disruption

ALTERNATIVE TREATMENTS

- extensor tendon repair
- distal interphalangeal fusion

MANAGEMENT

Stack Techniques
- Stack® splint
- closed pinning optional

POSTOPERATIVE MANAGEMENT

- 6 weeks of full-time splinting then
- 2 weeks nighttime splinting

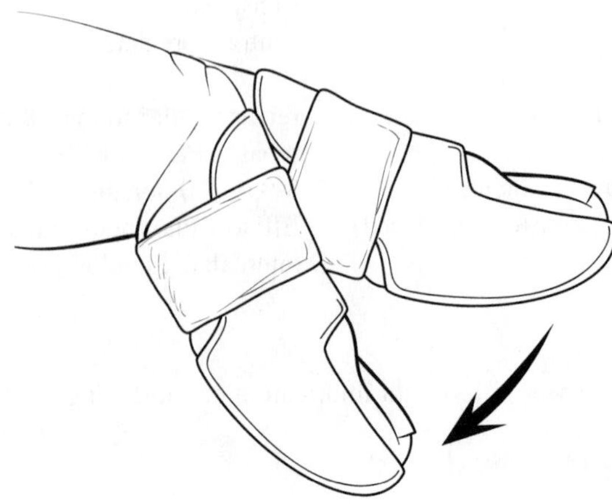

Splint DIP - allow PIP motion

REHABILITATION

- Proximal interphalangeal (PIP) motion exercises while distal interphalangeal is splinted

COMPLICATIONS

- higher complication rate when treated surgically
- skin maceration
- joint stiffness
- extensor lag

SELECTED REFERENCES

Schneider LH. Commentary. J Hand Surg 1993;18A:608.
Schneider LH. Fractures of the distal interphalangeal joint. Hand Clin 1994;10:277–285.
Wehbe MA, Schneider LH et al. Mallet fractures. J Bone Joint Surg 1984;66A:658–669.

NOTES

REPAIR OF MALLET FINGER

CPT code **26433 repair of extensor tendon, distal insertion, primary or secondary, without graft (e.g., mallet finger)**

ICD-9 code **736.1 mallet finger**

INDICATIONS

- failure of Stack® splint
- displaced intra-articular fragment
- joint subluxation

SURGICAL ANATOMY

- extensor tendon insertion on the distal phalanx

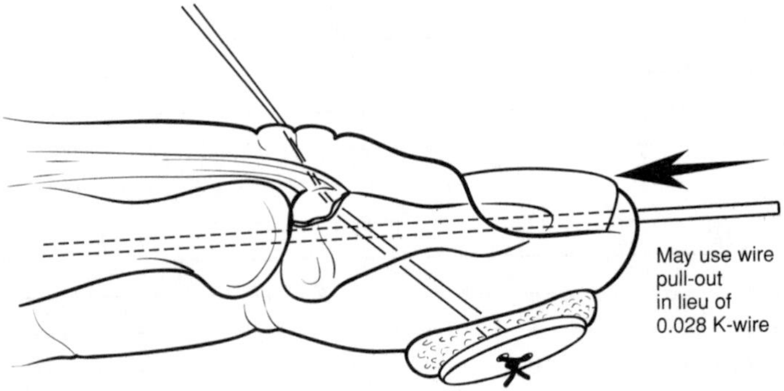

APPROACH

- transverse incision over DIP joint

Surgical Techniques

- clean fracture site with rongeur
- reduction of fragment using fluoroscopy
- place 0.028 K-wire against small fragment to buttress distally into reduced position
- place 0.035 K-wire through DIP to maintain distal phalanx reduction

POSTOPERATIVE MANAGEMENT

- hand-based splint
- remove pins after 4–6 weeks

REHABILITATION

- active range of motion following pin or pull-out wire removal

COMPLICATIONS

- extension lag
- DIP stiffness
- painful fragment nonunion

NOTES

RESECTION OF SUPERNUMERARY DIGIT

CPT code **26587 reconstruction of supernumerary digit, soft tissue and bone**

ICD-9 codes **755.07 polydactyly, foot**
755.04 polydactyly, hand
755.66 toe anomaly, congenital

INDICATIONS

- to enhance function and cosmesis for hand duplications
- facilitate shoe wear, and minimize discomfort in foot duplications
- see Wassel reference for classification

ALTERNATIVE TREATMENTS

- observation
- modifications of shoes (extra width)
- small skin tags may be tied off in the newborn nursery

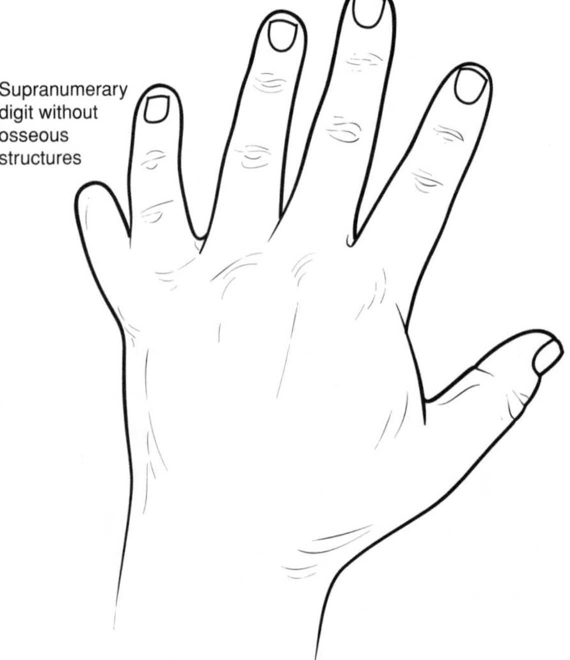

SURGICAL ANATOMY

Incision

- usually racket-shaped incision for border digit
- Bilhaut-Cloquet technique for distal phalanx of the thumb

APPROACHES

Surgical Techniques

- supine position, tourniquet control
- principles: maintain size, stability, motor control, vascularity, flexibility, web space depth, and strength
- usually excise border digit and preserve most functional digit
- preoperative x-rays: important to identify bony anatomy
- postaxial (little finger): racket incision, preserve vessels, re-attach collateral ligament, K-wire as needed
- preaxial (thumb): Wassel classification determines technique; ulnar digit usually is preserved
- skin grafting may be required

POSTOPERATIVE MANAGEMENT

- cast or hand dressing for 3–6 weeks followed by pin removal

REHABILITATION

- occupational therapy for range of motion

COMPLICATIONS

- infection <1%
- stiffness, instability of digit
- skin contracture, uncosmetic scar
- persistence of cartilaginous anlage

SELECTED REFERENCES

Wassel HD. The results of surgery for polydactyly of the thumb: a review. Clin Orthop 1969;64:175.

Tuch BA, Lipp EB, et al. A review of supernumerary thumb and its surgical management. Clin Orthop 1977;125:159.

METACARPAL FRACTURE, CLOSED TREATMENT

CPT code **26600 closed treatment of metacarpal fracture, single; without manipulation, each bone**

ICD-9 code **815.00 closed fracture of metacarpal bone(s)**

INDICATIONS

- treatment of nondisplaced and nonangulated (<10º) metacarpal diaphyseal fracture
- fracture of metaphysis will permit some additional angulation, particularly in the child
- Boxer's fracture with <30º angulation (4th or 5th distal metacarpal)

HAND

ALTERNATIVE TREATMENTS

- open reduction–internal fixation with plate or screws
- percutaneous fixation with K-wires
- use of Galveston metacarpal splint

ANATOMY

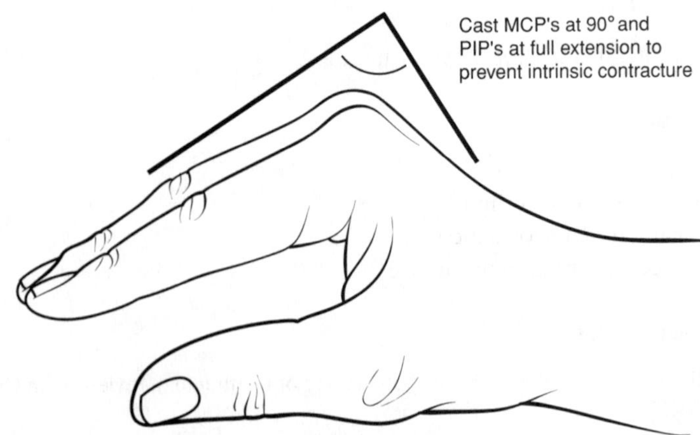

- proper rotational alignment is critical because even slight rotation will result in malalignment with the fingers in flexion
- metacarpal phalangeal (MCP) is a cam-joint, so every effort should be made to flex the MCPs and avoid collateral contracture
- extension of proximal interphalangeal joints also prevents intrinsic muscule contracture during healing

MANAGEMENT

- "buddy-tape" affected finger to adjacent finger to prevent rotation
- use gutter splint for fourth and fifth metacarpals; short arm cast or orthoplast splint for remaining bones

REHABILITATION

- begin active and passive range of motion of MCP once tenderness decreases (3–4 weeks)

COMPLICATIONS

- rotational deformity of mid-shaft fractures
- limited range of motion secondary to collateral or intrinsic tightness
- volar metacarpal head prominence on power grip with Boxer's fracture

NOTES

METACARPAL FRACTURE, OPEN TREATMENT

CPT code **26615 open treatment of metacarpal fracture, single, with or without internal or external fixation, each bone**

ICD-9 code **815.00 closed fracture of metacarpal bone(s)**

INDICATIONS

- shortened, angulated or comminuted fracture
- open fracture with fixation depending on nature of soft tissue injury

ALTERNATIVE TREATMENT

- closed treatment per 26600

SURGICAL ANATOMY

- use dorsal approach
- sweep extensor tendon sheath aside to expose bone

Surgical Techniques

- use of minifragment set (1.5 mm cortical screws and buttress plate)
- transverse fractures should generally be plated
- oblique fractures may be amenable to parallel K-wires

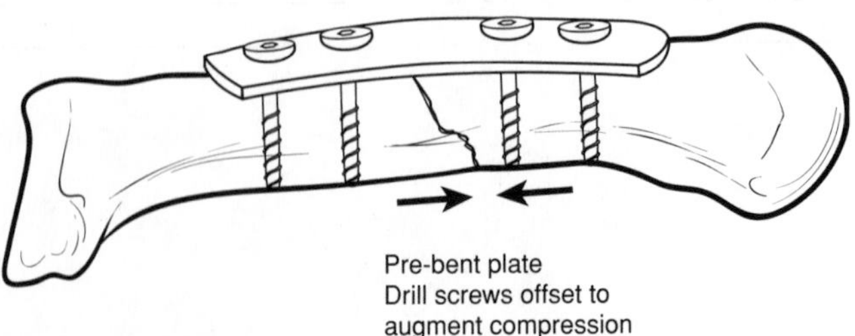

POSTOPERATIVE MANAGEMENT

- immobilize for 7–10 days
- begin active range of motion (fixation must be stable)

REHABILITATION

- same as for 26600

COMPLICATIONS

- infection
- loss of reduction and fixation
- extensor adhesions if plate is placed dorsally
- use smooth K-wires to prevent digital nerve injury

NOTES

PART VI

HIP

ADDUCTOR TENOTOMY, OBTURATOR NEURECTOMY

CPT code	**27003 tenotomy, adductor, subcutaneous, open, with obturator neurectomy**
ICD-9 codes	**343.9 infantile cerebral palsy, unspecified**
	781.2 abnormality of gait; gait: ataxic, paralytic

INDICATION

- hip subluxation and dislocation with contracture of adductor muscle

ALTERNATIVE TREATMENTS

- physical therapy, stretching, and range of motion
- bracing in hip abduction brace for nighttime and/or daytime
- myoneural blocks with 45% alcohol
- botox injection into adductor muscle to temporarily simulate effects of surgery

SURGICAL ANATOMY

Incision

- transverse (more cosmetic) or longitudinal; close to origin of adductor muscle near pubis

APPROACHES

Surgical Technique

- supine position; hip abducted and externally rotated
- transverse incision close to pubis, identify tendinous portion of muscle and release completely
- also, myotomy of proximal gracilis in independent ambulators
- anterior branch obturator neurectomy if patient also has scissoring
- adductor brevis myotomy (partial) if hips cannot be abducted more than 30–40° after other procedures (above)
- postoperative drain

POSTOPERATIVE MANAGEMENT

- abduction pillow
- hip spica cast, if not compliant

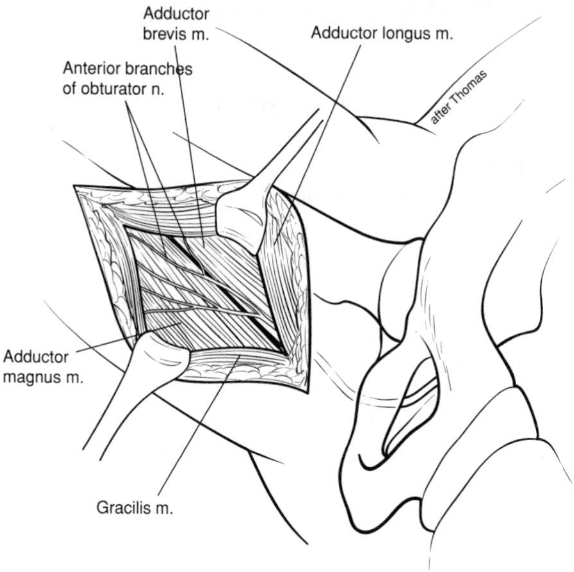

REHABILITATION

- range of motion and stretching; hip abduction pillow
- occasionally need hip spica cast for 3–4 weeks
- nighttime hip abduction brace for 6–12 months

COMPLICATIONS

- hip abduction contracture from overcorrection; can occur after anterior branch neurectomy
- further hip subluxation and dislocation
- infection
- hematoma

SELECTED REFERENCE

Bleck EE. Orthopaedic management in cerebral palsy. Philadelphia: JB Lippincott, 1987:286–296.

NOTES

HIP ARTHROTOMY FOR SEPSIS

CPT code **27030 arthrotomy, hip with drainage (e.g., infection)**

ICD-9 codes **711.05 pyogenic arthritis**
730.25 osteomyelitis, pelvis/hip

INDICATION

- septic arthritis of hip and/or osteomyelitis of proximal femur

ALTERNATIVE TREATMENTS

- hip arthroscopy (unproven record)
- intravenous antibiotics without arthrotomy (not recommended in hip)

SURGICAL ANATOMY

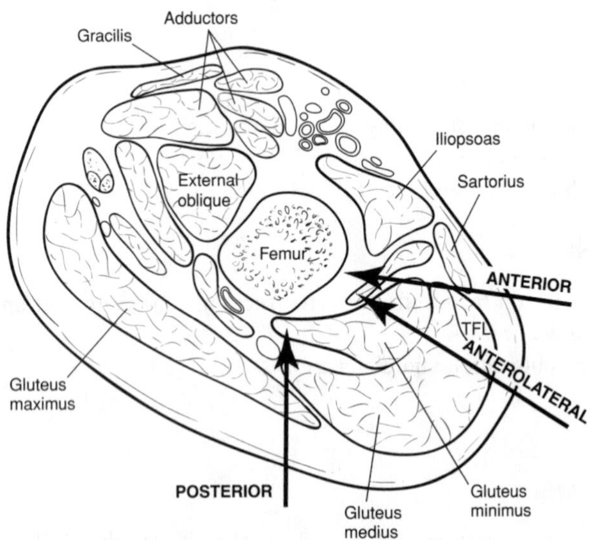

1. anterior approach via longitudinal or transverse (recommended) incision about one fingerbreadth below anterior superior iliac spine (ASIS)
2. anterolateral approach: Watson-Jones approach
3. posterior: more difficult; risk of sciatic nerve damage, compromise to hip blood supply (AVN), and higher dislocation rate, BUT promotes dependent drainage
4. medial: typically not used because of unfamiliar approach and risk of avascular necrosis (AVN)

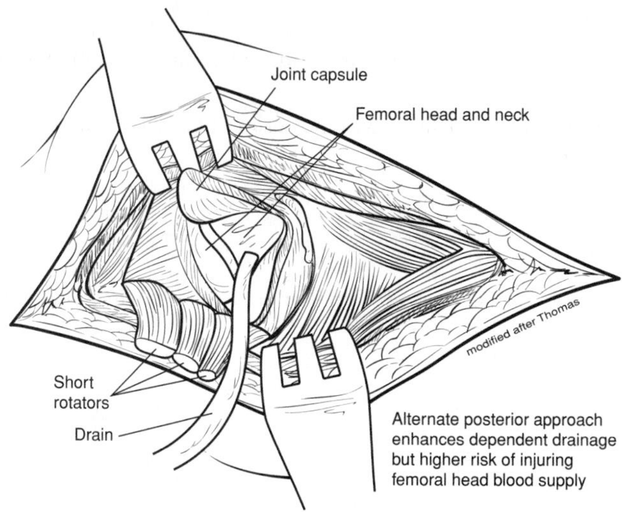

APPROACHES

Surgical Techniques (Anterior Approach)

- supine position.
- transverse incision about one fingerbreadth below ASIS
- identify and protect lateral femoral cutaneous nerve of thigh
- superficial surgical interval: sartorius and tensor fascia lata
- deep surgical interval: rectus femoris and gluteus medius
- capsulotomy. obtain cultures
- put catheter into hip joint and irrigate
- postoperative drain or Penrose
- loosely close wound but leave fascia open

POSTOPERATIVE MANAGEMENT

- pull drain on postoperative day 1 or 2
- intravenous antibiotics (duration per ID consultant)
- Motrin helpful for postoperative fever and pain
- occasionally requires second "wash-out" in operating room

REHABILITATION

- encourage hip range of motion
- crutches if older than 7 years; otherwise, wheelchair
- weight-bear as tolerated

COMPLICATIONS

- post-infectious arthritis, if not treated promptly (surgery within 24–36° of symptom onset)
- dislocation (mostly associated with posterior approach or neglected cases presenting late)
- AVN

SELECTED REFERENCE

Sucato DJ, Schwend RM, Gillespie R. Septic arthritis of the hip in children. J Am Acad Orthop Surg 1997;5:249–260.

NOTES

RESECTION ARTHROPLASTY, HIP

CPT code **27122 acetabuloplasty; resection, femoral head (e.g., Girdlestone's procedure)**

ICD-9 code(s)
711.06 chronic infection of the hip
996.66 infected total hip arthroplasty
996.4 unreconstructable failed total hip arthroplasty

INDICATIONS

- persistent infection about the hip, with recurrent abscesses or osteomyelitis of the proximal femur or acetabulum
- infected total hip arthroplasty or a failed total hip arthroplasty that is technically or practically unreconstructable

ALTERNATIVE TREATMENTS

- aggressive debridement, with removal of any involved bone
- irrigation, debridement, and synovectomy with acetabular liner exchange for an acute infection of a prosthetic hip
- one-stage revision, with component removal and reimplantation of an infected prosthetic hip
- revision total hip arthroplasty

SURGICAL ANATOMY

Incision
- anterolateral
- direct lateral
- posterolateral

APPROACHES

Surgical Techniques
- position: lateral decubitus
- incision: longitudinal (direct lateral) or posterior curved (posterolateral)
- incise iliotibial band (ITB)
- gluteal elevation (direct lateral) or division of short external rotators (posterolateral)
- femoral neck cut or removal of femoral implant (with or without femoral osteotomy) and debridement of proximal femur
- debridement of acetabulum or removal of acetabular component with reaming
- closure (primary vs delayed primary vs secondary depending upon patient and organism)

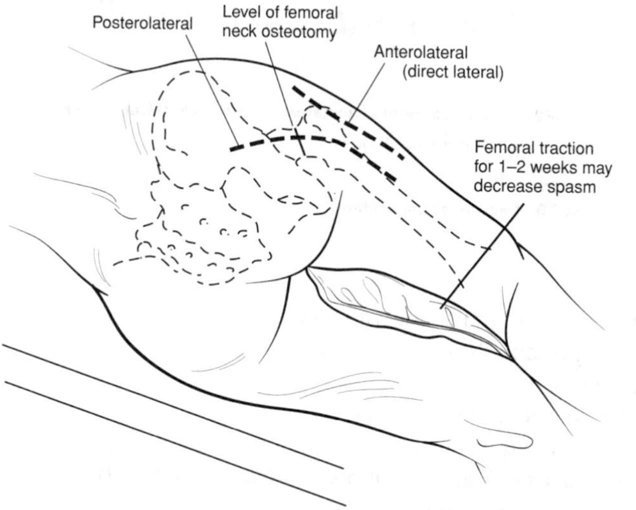

POSTOPERATIVE MANAGEMENT

- bedrest with or without skeletal traction on involved extremity to prevent painful proximal migration of the femoral head secondary to muscle spasm

REHABILITATION

- gradual mobilization at 3–4 weeks with walker; touch-down weight-bearing (TDWB) on affected extremity
- if Girdlestone is permanent, it may be able to bear partial weight comfortably on affected extremity with shoe lift (anticipate minimum of 4 months)

COMPLICATIONS

- recurrent infection
- neurologic injury about 1%
- leg length discepancy (all patients with permanent Girdlestone)
- deep venous thrombosis incidence (DVT) 50% overall; 3–9% proximal with prophylaxis

SELECTED REFERENCES

Bittar ES, Petty W. Girdlestone arthroplasty for infected total hip arthroplasty. Clin Orthop 1982;170:83.

Girdlestone GR. Acute pyogenic arthritis of the hip; operation giving free access and effective drainage. Lancet 1943;1:419.

CLOSED TREATMENT OF ACETABULAR FRACTURE

CPT code **27220 closed treatment of acetabulum (hip socket) fracture(s); without manipulation**

ICD-9 code **808.0 fracture of the acetabulum**

INDICATIONS

- acetabular fracture in patient with medical contraindication to surgery
- pre-existing osteoarthrosis of the involved hip
- local infection
- osteopenia of the inominate bone
- fracture(s) without displacement
- fracture with a small amount of posttraumatic incongruity
  - low transverse fracture
  - low anterior column fracture with <1–1.5-cm displacement
  - small posterior wall fragment (< 35–50% wall–stable in flexion)
- both column fracture achieving secondary congruity

ALTERNATIVE TREATMENTS

- open reduction–internal fixation
- acute total hip arthroplasty

REHABILITATION

- bedrest for 5 weeks
- active motion of the hip allowed during bedrest
- continuous passive motion of the knee and hip started 3 or 4 days posttrauma
- prophylactic anticoagulation during period of bedrest
- crutch or walker gait with progressive partial weight-bearing is allowed after 5–6 weeks

COMPLICATIONS

- displacement of the fracture with malunion
- development of posttraumatic osteoathritis of the hip
- deep venous thrombosis

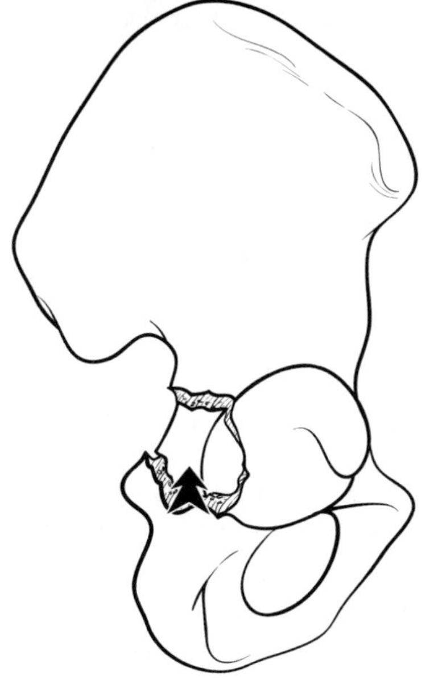

HIP

SELECTED REFERENCE

Letournel E, Judet R. General principles of management of acetabular fractures. In: Fractures of the acetabulum, 2nd ed. New York: Springer-Verlag, 1993:347–359.

NOTES

FEMORAL NECK FRACTURE

CPT code **27235 percutaneous skeletal fixation of femoral fracture, proximal end, neck, nondisplaced, mildly displaced, or impacted fracture**

ICD-9 codes **733.14 pathologic fracture of neck of femur**
820 fracture of neck of femur
820.03 base of neck; cervicotrochanteric section

INDICATIONS

- impacted or nondisplaced (Garden type I or II), intracapsular fractures of the femoral neck
- Garden II/Pauwels III (with vertical fracture angle) may be more appropriately considered with Garden III (displaced) fractures

ALTERNATIVE TREATMENTS

- nonoperative treatment in patients with stable fractures and minimal pain on physical examination or in nonambulatory patients
- pinning with capsulotomy or joint aspiration to prevent intracapsular pressure and distention as prophylaxis against osteonecrosis

SURGICAL ANATOMY

Incision

- direct lateral, just distal to vastus tubercle, extending approximately 4 cm, *or*
- 3 stab incisions (for each screw)

APPROACHES

Surgical Techniques

- supine, hemilithotomy position on fracture table
- before incision: fluoroscopic examination to confirm fracture impaction and stability
- internally rotate hip to prevent posterior displacement of the femoral head and to place the femoral neck parallel to the floor
- incise iliotibial band (ITB) and vastus lateralis
- 3 parallel, cannulated 7.3-mm hip screws, triangular configuration, starting approximately 2.5–3.0 cm below vastus tubercle, angled at 135–150° from the femoral shaft
- starting point should *not* be distal to the lesser trochanter
- "long lag" screws may cross the fracture to improve purchase in osteopenic bone, if there is adequate fracture compression

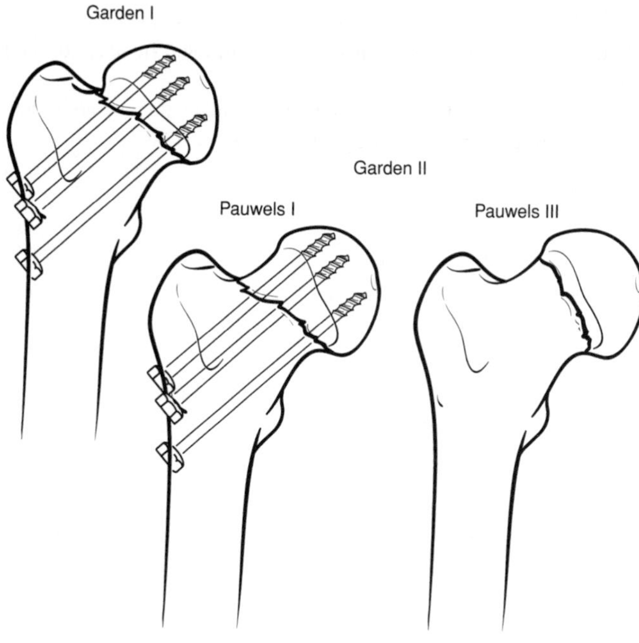

- fluoroscopic examination with hip rotation to confirm fracture stability and ensure screws do not penetrate joint

POSTOPERATIVE MANAGEMENT

- deep venous thrombosis (DVT) prophylaxis
- osteopenic bone workup and management

REHABILITATION

- touch-down weight-bearing (severe osteopenia, nonimpacted fractures)
- weight-bearing as tolerated (WBAT) (stable, impacted fractures)

COMPLICATIONS

- non-union <5%
- osteonecrosis <7–10%
- screw "cut out" or penetration into hip joint
- DVT >50% with no prophylaxis
- the 9 "Ds": dehydration, delirium, dementia, depression, dietary deficiencies, deconditioning, decubitus ulcers, drug effects, and death (mortality during the first postoperative year is 20% for the elderly)

SELECTED REFERENCES

Garden RS. Malreduction and avascular necrosis in subcapital fractures of the femur. J Bone Joint Surg Br 1971;53:183.

Koval KJ, Kuckerman JD. Hip fractures: I. Overview and evaluation and treatment of femoral–neck fractures. J Am Acad Orthop Surg 1994;2:141–149.

NOTES

DISPLACED FEMORAL NECK FRACTURE

CPT code **27236 open treatment of femoral fracture, proximal end, neck, internal fixation or prosthetic replacement (direct fracture exposure)**

ICD-9 codes **733.14 pathologic fracture of neck of femur**
820.00 intracapsular section, unspecified

INDICATIONS

- displaced (Garden types III and IV) fractures of the femoral neck
- young, active patients require immediate open reduction–internal fixation and pinning
- older, less active patients require hemiarthroplasty after medical stabilization

ALTERNATIVE TREATMENTS

- closed reduction and pinning
- basilar neck fractures may require open reduction–internal fixation with sliding compression hip screw and parallel derotation screw
- total hip arthroplasty in patients with significant, pre-existing, symptomatic arthritis
- nonoperative treatment in the debilitated, nonambulatory patient, although chronic pain is problematic
- Girdlestone resection of femoral head, if infection is present

SURGICAL ANATOMY

Incision

- direct lateral for open reduction-internal fixation
- anterolateral or posterolateral for hemiarthroplasty

APPROACHES

Surgical Technique: open reduction-internal fixation

- lateral decubitus position preferred to allow hip range of motion
- supine, hemilithotomy position on fracture table is possible and allows easier fluoroscopic views
- reduction by flexion, slight traction, internal rotation, and then abduction
- incision: direct lateral
- incise iliotibial band (ITB), split vastus lateralis in continuity with inferior fibers of gluteus medius
- capsulotomy in line with femoral neck for direct fracture exposure

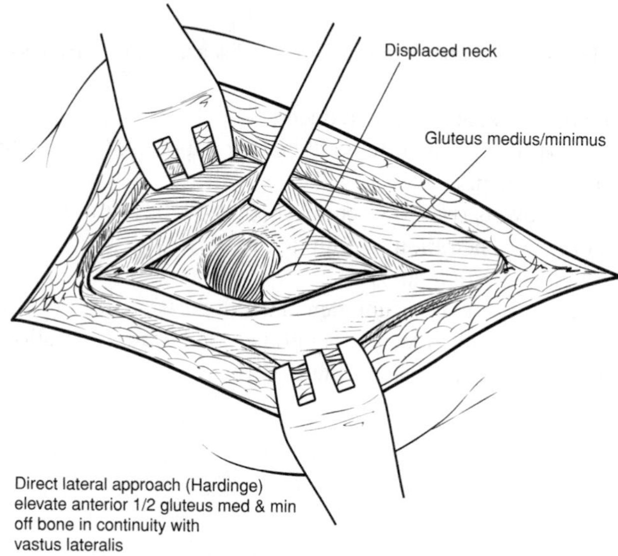

- 3 parallel, cannulated 7.3-mm hip screws placed in triangular configuration (refer to technique described for CPT code 27235)
- consider bone graft
- *anatomic* reduction is critical to success!

Surgical Technique: Hemiarthroplasty

- lateral decubitus position
- follow exposure for total hip arthroplasty
- measure head circumference for unipolar (if between sizes, oversize to next 1 mm)
- femoral broaching
- component trialing
- cemented femoral component fixation preferred

POSTOPERATIVE MANAGEMENT

- DVT prophylaxis
- osteopenic bone workup and management

REHABILITATION

- open reduction–internal fixation: touch-down weight-bearing, no abductor exercise
- hemiarthroplasty: WBAT
- early mobility important

COMPLICATIONS

- *beware* of fractures secondary to metastatic disease (especially lesser trochanter)
- non-union <10%, if anatomically reduced
- osteonecrosis with subsequent femoral head collapse <33%, if anatomically reduced within 24 hours
- "high angle" (Pauwels type 3) fractures are more likely to fail
- screw "cut out" or penetration into hip joint
- DVT >50% with no prophylaxis
- the 9 "Ds": dehydration, delirium, dementia, depression, dietary deficiencies, deconditioning, decubitus ulcers, drug effects, and death (mortality for the first postoperative year is 20% for the elderly)

NOTES

EXTRACAPSULAR HIP FRACTURE

CPT code **27244** **open treatment of intertrochanteric, pertrochantic, or subtrochanteric femoral fracture; with plate or screw type implant, with or without cerclage**

ICD-9 codes **820.2** **intertrochanteric section**
820.22 **subtrochanteric section**

INDICATION

- mandatory open reduction–internal fixation to allow best chance of restoration of anatomic function and mobility

ALTERNATIVE TREATMENTS

- intramedullary reconstruction nail may be indicated for intertrochanteric fractures with significant subtrochanteric extension, reverse obliquity fractures, or high subtrochanteric fractures
- nonoperative treatment for nondisplaced or stress intertrochanteric fractures
- calcar replacement hemiarthroplasty may be considered in cases of severe osteopenia to allow early WBAT but usually is a salvage procedure for failed open reduction–internal fixation.

SURGICAL ANATOMY

Incision
- direct lateral approach to proximal femur, extending distally from vastus tubercle

APPROACHES

Surgical Techniques
- position: supine, hemilithotomy on fracture table
- closed reduction with traction and internal rotation under fluoroscopy; femoral neck parallel to the floor for easy orientation
- longitudinal direct lateral incision
- split ITB
- split vastus lateralis posteriorly
- angled compression hip screw for routine intertrochanteric fractures; consider 95° screw or blade plate for fractures with significant subtrochanteric extension
- cannulated guide pin, *avoiding varus*; tip of pin should be *central* in the femoral head or slightly inferior and posterior
- ream

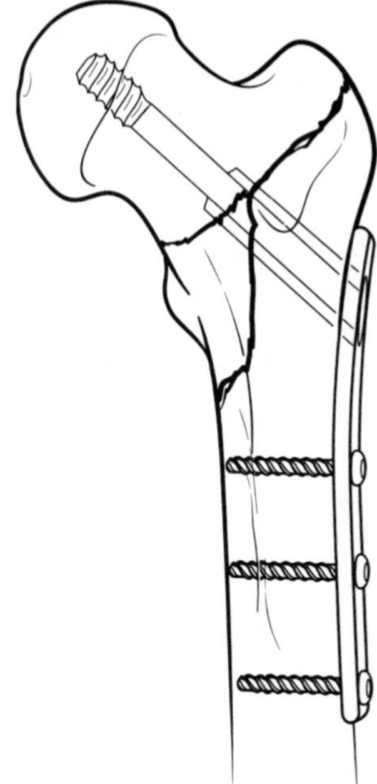

- place compression screw, assemble, and attach sideplate, typically 6–8 cortices below distal end of fracture
- cerclage or lag screw postcromedial buttress (lesser trochanter) when possible
- avoid surgical stripping medially to preserve bone vascularity
- assess rotational stability and hardware placement
- closure

POSTOPERATIVE MANAGEMENT

- DVT prophylaxis
- assessment and management of osteopenic bone

REHABILITATION

- touch-down weight-bearing for unstable fractures, WBAT for stable fractures with solid fixation

COMPLICATIONS

- *beware* of fractures secondary to metastatic disease
- loss of fixation 10–20%; related to osteopenia, improper hardware position, or loss of fixation of posteromedial buttress

- DVT >50% with no prophylaxis
- the 9 "Ds": dehydration, delirium, dementia, depression, dietary deficiencies, deconditioning, decubitus ulcers, drug effects, and death (mortality during the first postoperative year is 20% for the elderly)

SELECTED REFERENCES

Baumgaertner MR. Awareness of the tip-apex distance reduces failure of fixation of trochanteric fractures of the hip. J Bone Joint Surg Br 1997;79(6):969.

Koval KJ, Zuckerman JD. Hip fractures: II. Evaluation and treatment of intertrochanteric fractures. J Am Acad Orthop Surg 1994;2:150–156.

NOTES

INTRAMEDULLARY RODDING OF INTER- OR SUBTROCHANTERIC FRACTURE

CPT code **27245** **open treatment of intertrochanteric, pertrochanteric, or subtrochanteric femoral fracture with intramedullary implant, with or without interlocking screws or cerclage**

ICD-9 codes **820.22** **subtrochanteric fracture (open, 820.32)**
733.15 **pathologic fracture**
733.20 **cyst of bone**

INDICATIONS

- closed, open, or pathologic pertrochanteric or subtrochanteric femur fracture in an otherwise stable patient
- impending pathologic fracture

ALTERNATIVE TREATMENTS

- traction immobilization
- radiation therapy (pathologic lesion)
- sliding screw and plate fixation
- blade plate and screw fixation
- prosthetic replacement

SURGICAL ANATOMY

APPROACH

- direct lateral

Surgical Techniques

- equipment: fracture table, fluoroscope
- position: supine on fracture table or lateral on beanbag
- fracture reduction performed
- incision: tip of greater trochanter, extending 6–8 mm proximally and posteriorly
- gluteus maximus split inline
- piriformis fossa identified
- starting position confirmed in anteroposterior and lateral views
- proximal femur opened
- ball tip guide wire inserted
- femur reamed, fracture held reduced

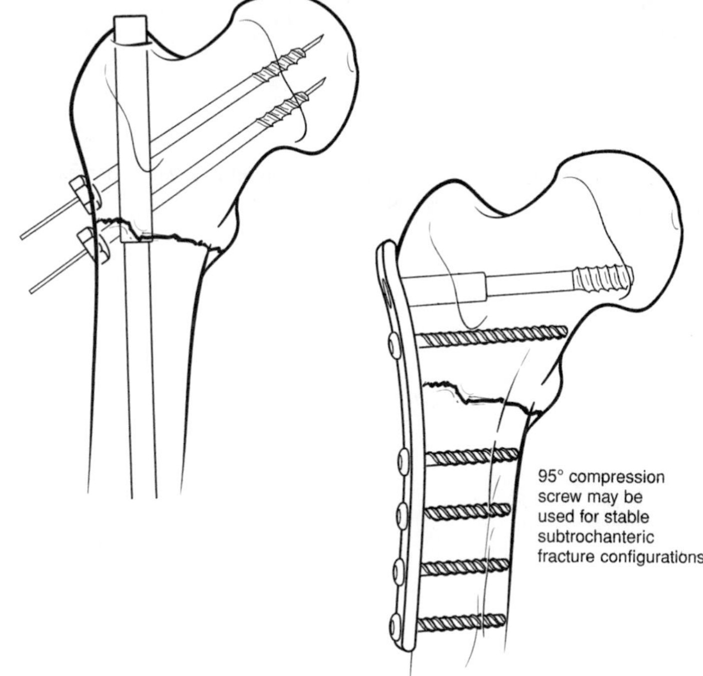

- length and diameter determined
- guidewire exchanged for smooth tip
- nail inserted
- locking screws inserted as needed
- final imaging
- closure

POSTOPERATIVE MANAGEMENT

- DVT prophylaxis

REHABILITATION

- weight-bearing based on stability
- immediate range of motion for hip, knee, and ankle
- gait training as indicated

COMPLICATIONS

- loss of fixation
- non-union

- malunion
- infection
- DVT

SELECTED REFERENCE

Wiss DA, Brien WW. Subtrochanteric fractures of the femur: results of treatment by interlocking nailing. Clin Orthop 1992;283:231–236.

NOTES

HIP DISLOCATION

CPT code	**27252 closed treatment of hip dislocation, traumatic; requiring anesthesia**
ICD-9 codes	**835.01 closed posterior dislocation of hip**
	835.03 closed anterior dislocation of hip

INDICATIONS

- traumatic hip dislocation is an orthopaedic emergency; the incidence of osteonecrosis and neurovascular compromise increases significantly with delay of reduction

ALTERNATIVE TREATMENTS

- gentle closed reduction with sedation should first be attempted in the emergency room
- open reduction, if closed treatment not successful or concentric reduction is not achieved

SURGICAL ANATOMY

- anterior: 10%; femoral head may compress femoral neurovascular bundle; head fracture or indentation likely
  - superior: result from abduction, external rotation, and hyperextension force
  - inferior (more common): result from abduction, external rotation, and flexion force
- posterior: 90%; classified by Epstein on the basis of femoral head, neck, or acetabular fracture; femoral head may compress the sciatic nerve; superior gluteal neurvovascular injury may occur; result from force applied to flexed knee along femur axis
  - simple: with hip in neutral or adducted position
  - with acetabular fracture: hip in abducted position

Incision

- only if closed reduction attempt fails, reduction is nonconcentric on x-ray, or associated fracture requires open reduction–internal fixation

APPROACHES

- anterior dislocation: closed reduction by traction, then extension/adduction and internal rotation (see description, p. 171)
- posterior dislocation: closed reduction by traction, then flexion/adduction and external rotation
- second assistant provides counter-traction force against ilium
- assess stability through range of motion
- postreduction anteroposterior, frog lateral, and Judet views of the acetabulum are mandatory; computed tomography of the hip joint to rule out incarcerated fragment
- fragments involving less than 25% of the posterior wall of the acetabulum usually do not affect stability, those involving 25–50% need to be carefully examined, and those involving over 50% are unstable and need to be repaired surgically

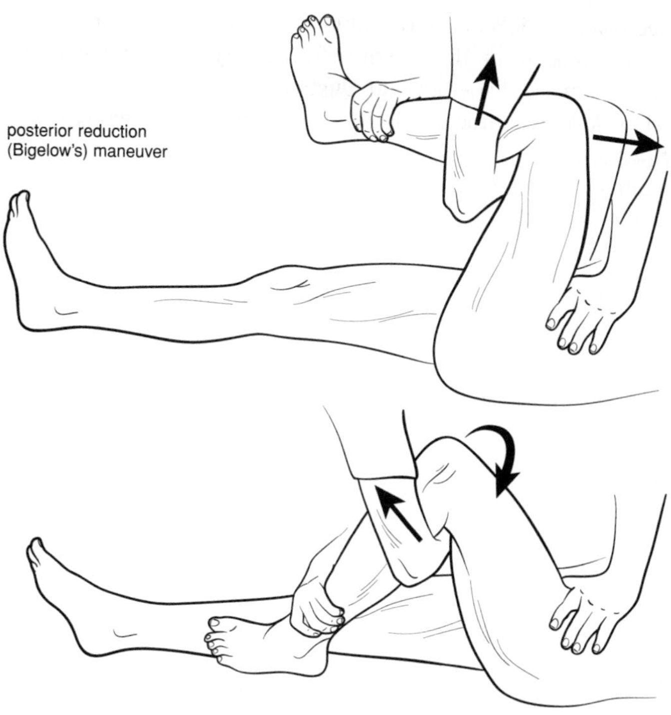

Surgical Techniques

- dictated by the position of dislocation and associated fracture
- sizeable intra-articular osteochondral fragments or compression fractures require joint exploration and excision or internal fixation

POSTOPERATIVE MANAGEMENT

- neurovascular examination
- DVT prophylaxis

REHABILITATION

- Weight-bearing depends on the stability of the hip and presence of associated fractures

COMPLICATIONS

- osteonecrosis, 10–50%; usually within 2 years but can occur up to 5 years after injury; depends on the severity of the injury, delay in reduction >6 hours, or repeated attempts at reduction
- femoral neck or head fracture during reduction; forceful reductions should not be performed
- degenerative arthritis

SELECTED REFERENCE

Epstein HC. Traumatic dislocation hip. Baltimore: Williams & Wilkins, 1980.

NOTES

TOTAL HIP DISLOCATION, CLOSED REDUCTION

CPT code **27265 closed treatment of post hip arthroplasty dislocation; without anesthesia**

ICD-9 codes **996.66 due to internal joint prosthesis**
996.4 mechanical complication of internal orthopedic device

INDICATIONS

- traumatic or atraumatic dislocation
- contraindicated with component dissociation, dislocation of constrained acetabular component, or possible subluxation of acetabular component during perioperative period

ALTERNATIVE TREATMENTS

- closed reduction under anesthesia
- open reduction with or without component revision

SURGICAL ANATOMY

- essential to assess etiology of dislocation
  - acetabular abduction and anteversion
  - femoral anteversion

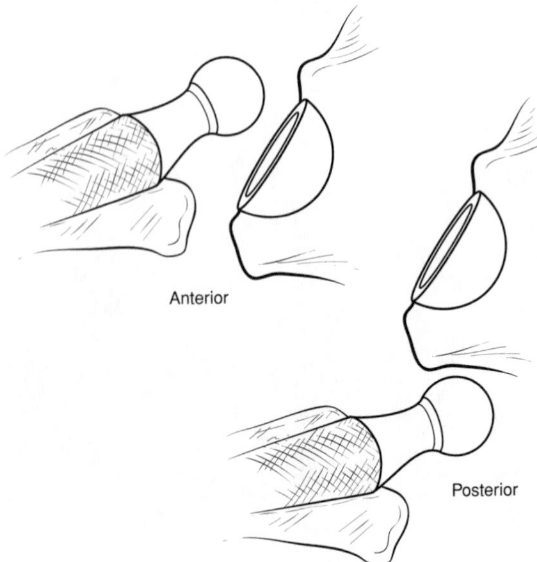

- need AP and shoot-thru lateral x-rays

  - leg length
  - altered soft tissue tension, e.g., hip center offset
  - evidence of component impingement
- assess direction of dislocation: anterior or posterior (superior unusual without significant cup abduction)

Techniques
- use conscious sedation to ensure adequate patient relaxation
- for posterior dislocation, use Bigelow's maneuver (see hip dislocation CPT 27252)
- for anterior dislocation, use Leadbetter's maneuver (flex to 90° with internal rotation followed by traction and circumduction into abduction in internal rotation with hip extension); or if adequately relaxed, direct inline traction with slight adduction in external rotation followed by internal rotation and abduction

POSTOPERATIVE MANAGEMENT

- if possible, fluoroscopically examine postreduction to establish "safe" range of motion
- place patient in abduction orthosis
- follow-up in 1–2 weeks postreduction once patient can ambulate without significant pain

REHABILITATION

- it is essential that the total hip not redislocate until adequate soft tissue healing and stability are achieved
- if dislocation occurs within the first 6 weeks of surgery due to mal-positioning of the hip by patient and there are no predisposing issues (see anatomy above), recurrent dislocation is unusual
- if dislocation occurs after 3 months or the patient experiences recurrent dislocation, long-term use of an abduction orthosis will be necessary due to high likelihood of recurrent dislocation

COMPLICATIONS

- recurrent dislocation
- soft tissue interposition preventing reduction
- dislodgement of uncemented acetabular component, if perioperative
- neuropraxia (rare)

PART VII

KNEE

KNEE ARTHROTOMY

CPT code	**27310**	**arthrotomy, knee, with exploration, drainage, or removal of foreign body (e.g., infection)**
ICD-9 codes	**711.06**	**septic knee joint**
	891.1	**loose body in knee joint**

INDICATIONS

- failure of septic knee to resolve despite repeated aspiration or arthroscopic lavage
- symptomatic foreign body that cannot be removed arthroscopically

ALTERNATIVE TREATMENTS

- infection
  - serial aspirations (abandon if reaccumulated volume or WBC count not decreased after 24–36°)
  - arthroscopic lavage with or without synovectomy
- foreign body
  - symptomatic and not retrievable by other means (i.e., arthroscopy)

SURGICAL ANATOMY

Incision

- anterior
- posterolateral
- posteromedial

APPROACHES

Surgical Techniques

- position: supine with tourniquet elevated (do not exsanguinate in presence of infection)
- incision: longitudinal midline
- arthrotomy: medial parapatellar
  - with or without lateral release to faciliate eversion of the patella
  - obtain multiple deep cultures
  - copious irrigation (≥9 L)

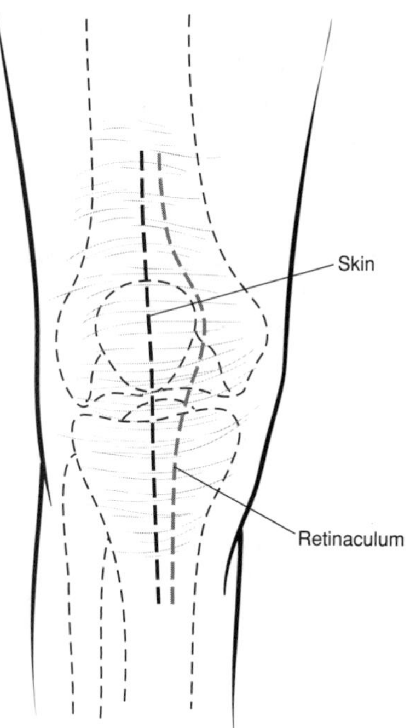

- usually with meticulous synovectomy
- placement of deep and superficial drains
- closure of medial capsule and skin (primary or delayed primary closure)

POSTOPERATIVE MANAGEMENT

- drains removed at 24–72 hours
- repeat arthrotomy, irrigation, and debridement with clinical suspicion of continued infection
- treatment with intravenous antibiotics specific for the infecting organism

REHABILITATION

- early (24–48 hours) active range of motion
- weight-bearing as tolerated, with crutches or walker for support

COMPLICATIONS

- persistent infection with chronic draining sinus
- bacteria-induced chondrolysis (especially Staphylococcus aureus)
- postinfectious degenerative joint disease

SELECTED REFERENCES

Ballard E, Burkhalter WE, Mayfield GW, et al. The functional treatment of pyogenic arthritis of the adult knee. J Bone Joint Surg 1975;57A:1119.

Stanitsky CL, Harvell JC, Fu FH. Arthroscopy in acute septic knees: management in pediatric patients. Clin Orthop 1989;241:209.

Thiery JA. Arthroscopic drainage in septic arthridites of the knee: a multicenter study. J Arthosc Rel Surg 1989;5:65.

NOTES

EXCISION PREPATELLAR BURSA

CPT code **27340 excision, prepatellar bursa**

ICD-9 code **726.65 prepatellar bursitis**

INDICATIONS

- recurrent symptomatic prepatellar bursitis despite nonoperative treatment including nonsteroidal anti-inflammatory drugs, aspiration, steroid injection, and avoidance of kneeling
- failure of bursal healing after I&D for pyogenic bursitis

ALTERNATIVE TREATMENTS

- repeat aspiration or injection
- protective knee padding
- avoidance of kneeling

SURGICAL ANATOMY

Incision

- transverse over patella (in Langer's lines—more cosmetic)
- straight longitudinal at midline (any preexisting knee arthritis)

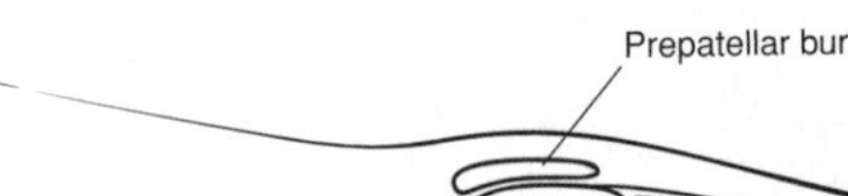

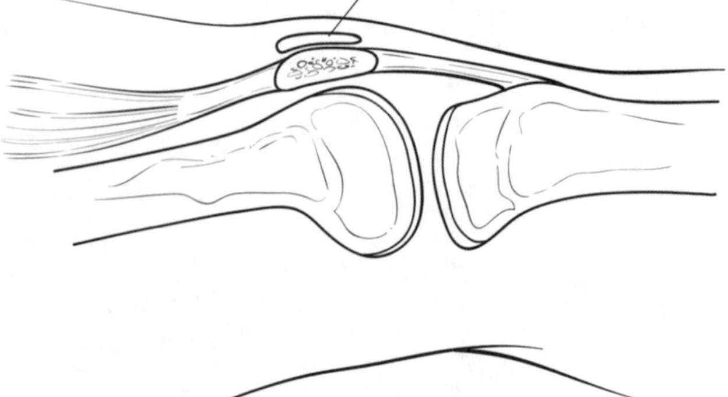

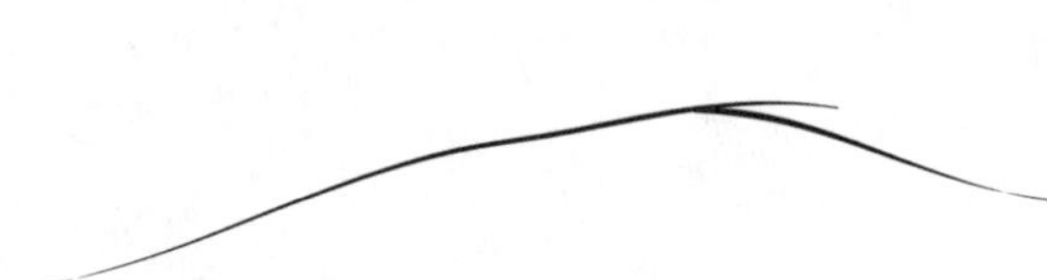

APPROACHES

Surgical Technique

- dissection of bursa (excise *in toto*)
- obliterate dead space
- with or without drain

POSTOPERATIVE MANAGEMENT

- compressive bandage
- knee immobilizer for 2 or 3 weeks

REHABILITATION

- quad sets
- straight leg raises
- begin range of motion at 1–2 weeks

COMPLICATIONS

- hematoma
- infection
- recurrent bursal distention

SELECTED REFERENCE

Phillips B. Non-traumatic disorders of joints. In: Crenshaw AH, ed. Campbell's operative orthopaedics, 8th ed. Baltimore: CV Mosby, 1992:1945–1946.

NOTES

REPAIR OF QUADRICEPS RUPTURE

CPT code **27385 suture of quadriceps or hamstring muscle rupture; primary**

ICD-9 codes **727.6 rupture of tendon, nontraumatic**
727.65 quadriceps tendon

INDICATIONS

- two subgroups of patients with quadriceps rupture
  - "weekend warrior" male in his 30s or 40s
  - older, atraumatic, especially in patients with diabetes or steroid use
- surgical repair for significant extensor lag
- low threshold for repair: neglected ruptures requiring late repair have high failure rates

ALTERNATIVE TREATMENTS

- cast or brace in extension for 6 weeks
  - residual extensor lag or rerupture a risk

SURGICAL ANATOMY

- subcutaneous repair

APPROACHES

- use medial parapatellar approach
- *avoid* infrapatellar "smile" incision
  due to risk of skin necrosis with subsequent procedures

Surgical Techniques

- expose rupture including retinacular extension, if any
- place 3 longitudinal drill holes in patella, starting point at midpoint of superior surface
- place 2 no. 2 nonresorbable Krackow or modified Kessler sutures in quadriceps fascia; pass inner limb of each through central drill hole and outer limbs through peripheral holes
- reinforce with resorbable suture or, if necessary, use no. 5 nonresorbable cerclage suture
- repair retinaculum with no. 0 nonresorbable suture
- routine subcutaneous and skin closure

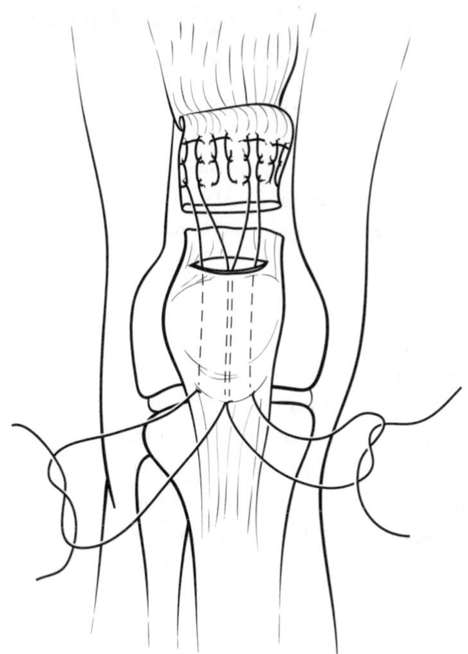

POSTOPERATIVE MANAGEMENT

- Robert Jones dressing with side splints for 7–10 days
- polycentric hinged brace (full length cuff) with 0–15° of motion for 6 weeks

REHABILITATION

- progressive range of motion based on knee motion
- begin straight leg raising exercise after first week
- active, gravity-assisted knee flexion after 6 weeks
- advance to isotonic or isokinetic strengthening at 6–12 weeks

COMPLICATIONS

- rerupture, especially in atraumatic patients
- residual extensor lag
- patella alta related to repair with altered patellofemoral mechanics

REPAIR OF TORN COLLATERAL LIGAMENT, KNEE

CPT code **27405 repair, primary, torn ligament, and/or capsule, knee; collateral**

ICD-9 codes **844 sprains and strains of knee and leg**
844.0 lateral collateral ligament of knee
844.1 medial collateral ligament of knee

INDICATIONS

- medial collateral ligament will heal with conservative care in cases of grade I (sprain) and II (some joint opening but an endpoint to valgus stress) injuries; consider reconstruction when associated with other ligamentous injuries and when complete (grade III: no endpoint to valgus stress)
- traumatic lateral collateral ligamentous injuries are often associated with knee dislocations and should be considered for early operative intervention; lateral collateral ligamentous attenuation injuries are often associated with chronic cruciate deficiencies and treated surgically after failure of bracing and activity modification

ALTERNATIVE TREATMENTS

- medial collateral ligament: casting (immediately after injury) and bracing
- lateral collateral ligament: casting and bracing

SURGICAL ANATOMY

- medial collateral ligament originates on the medial epicondyle and runs in a slightly anterior direction to the insertion 5–6 cm distal to the joint line
- lateral collateral ligament originates on the femoral epicondyle and passes just anterior and proximal to the popliteus with insertion into the fibular head

Incision

- depends on associated conditions being cared for and grafts necessary for reconstructions, but direct approach is preferred

APPROACH

Surgical Technique

- direct repair in traumatic situations and when bony avulsions exist; usually easier and better result when femoral attachment avulsed or injured

POSTOPERATIVE MANAGEMENT

- cast or brace for 1–2 weeks in slight flexion

REHABILITATION

- protected range of motion for 6–8 weeks
- avoid varus or valgus stress for 3 months
- sports at 6–9 months

COMPLICATIONS

- arthrofibrosis
- nerve injury: saphenous and peroneal

SELECTED REFERENCES

Gollehon DL, Torzilli PA, Warren RF. The role of the posterolateral and cruciate ligaments in stability of the human knee: a biomechanical study. J Bone Joint Surg 1987;69A:233–242.

Noyes F, Barber-Westin S. Surgical restoration to treat chronic deficiency of the posterolateral complex and cruciate ligaments of the knee joint. Am J Surg Med 1996;24:415–426.

Shelbourne KD, Porter DA. ACL-MCL injury: a preliminary report. Am J Surg Med 1992;20:283.

Warren LF, Marshall JL. The supporting structures and layers on the medial side of the knee. J Bone Joint Surg 1979;61A:56–62.

TIBIAL TUBERCLE OSTEOTOMY

CPT code **27418 anterior tibial tubercleplasty (e.g., Maquet type procedure)**

ICD-9 codes **717.7 chondromalacia patella**
836.3 dislocation of patella

INDICATIONS

- lateral facet osteoarthritis (Outerbridge type III or IV)
- failure of conservative treatment including vastus medialis obliquus strengthening, retinacular mobilization, and taping or bracing
- anteriomedialization for tracking malalignment requiring biplanar transposition

ALTERNATIVE TREATMENTS

- conservative treatment, as above
- static correction: traditional Elmslie-Trillat or other medialization surgeries
- dynamic correction: vastus medialis obliquus (VMO) or retinacular advancement
- (possibly) patellofemoral arthroplasty for advanced osteoarthritis (OA)

SURGICAL ANATOMY

- surgical anatomy is subcutaneous
- avoid vascular injury of anterior compartment during anteromedialization

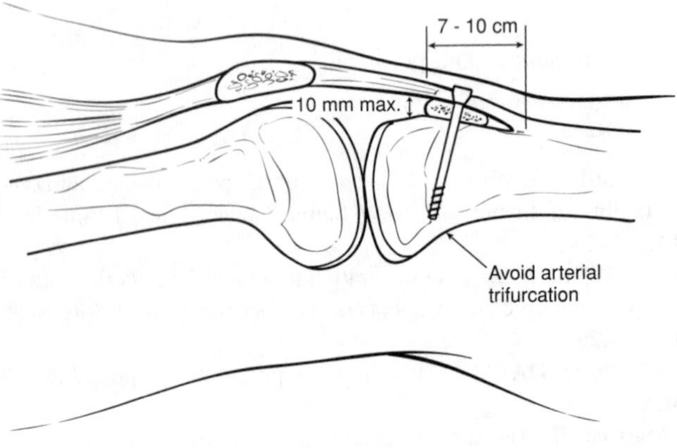

APPROACHES

- there are 2 primary approaches
  - direct anteriorization (Maquet)
  - anteromedialization (Fulkerson)
- maximum anteriorization of approximately 1 cm to avoid skin embarrassment
- single-cut anteromedialization requires careful planning to assess slope of tibial cut

POSTOPERATIVE MANAGEMENT

- immediate immobilization in Robert Jones dressing with splints
- begin active and gravity-assisted range of motion at 1 week
- protected partial weight-bearing for 6 weeks
- continue VMO strengthening throughout treatment

REHABILITATION

- results are contingent on maintaining quadriceps strength and balance

COMPLICATIONS

- persistent pain
- difficulty in kneeling or tenderness over tibial tubercle
- fracture at osteotomy, if too short or elevation too great
- inadequate medialization

SELECTED REFERENCE

Post WR, Fulkerson JP. Distal realignment of the patellofemoral joint. Indications, effects, results, and recommendations. Orthop Clin North Am 1992;23(4):631–643.

NOTES

REPAIR OF PATELLAR DISLOCATION

CPT code **27420 reconstruction of dislocating patella (e.g., Hauser type procedure)**

ICD-9 codes **717.7 chondromalacia of patella**
718.36 recurrent dislocation of patellofemoral joint

INDICATIONS

- recurrent patellar dislocation
- soft tissue or bony malalignment repair

ALTERNATIVE TREATMENTS

- conservative vastus medialis obliquus (VMO) strengthening, bracing, and retinacular mobilization
- isolated soft tissue repair with VMO and retinacular reefing

SURGICAL ANATOMY

- whether to perform dynamic or static reconstruction depends on assessment of deformity
  - increased quadriceps-angle or significant external tibial torsion suggests need for distal bony procedure
  - recurrent dislocation with deficit in medializing forces suggests use of VMO reefing

APPROACHES

- avoid Hauser's (sic) procedure, which medializes the tibial tubercle but also translates it posteriorly and increases patellofemoral stresses
- anteromedialization (Bandi or Elmslie-Trillat procedure) realigns distally but does not unload the arthritic patella to the same extent as Fulkerson's procedure
- Roux-Goldthwait (out of favor) uses the medial half of the patellar tendon to create a medializing sling for the lateral half of the tendon
- vastus medialis advancement involves translating the VMO insertion and using pants-over-vest imbrication sutures

POSTOPERATIVE MANAGEMENT

- long leg Robert Jones with side splints for 1 week
- soft tissue reconstruction: protected repair (active or gravity-assisted range of motion) for 6 weeks
- tibial tubercleplasty: protect until fracture healing has occurred (6–8 weeks)

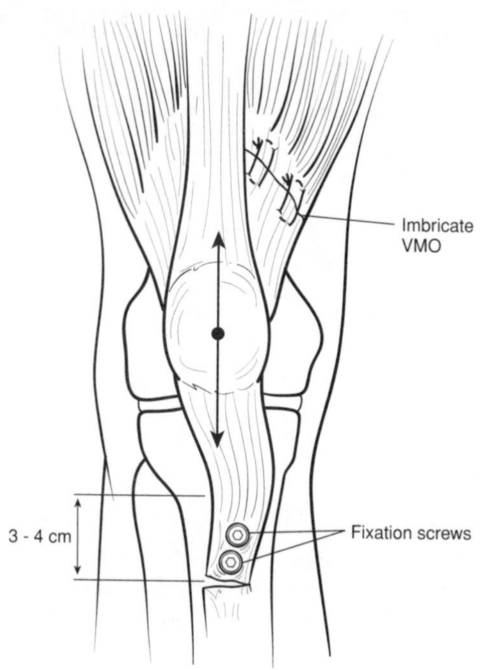

REHABILITATION

- begin isometric quadriceps strengthening immediately (straight leg raising)
- begin quadriceps isotonic or isokinetic strengthening at 6 weeks
- weight-bearing is delayed until fracture healing is complete in osteotomies

COMPLICATIONS

- inadequate realignment and recurrent dislocation
- overtightening of soft tissue repair and overload of patellofemoral joint
- osteoarthritis of the patellofemoral joint with inadequate anteriorization (Hauser's procedure)
- non-union of osteotomy (rare)

SELECTED REFERENCE

Fulkerson JP. Disorders of the patellofemoral joint. Baltimore: Williams & Wilkins, 1997.

CLOSED TREATMENT OF PATELLAR FRACTURE

CPT code **27520 closed treatment of patellar fracture, without manipulation**

ICD-9 codes **822 fracture of patella**
822.0 closed

INDICATIONS

- nondisplaced patellar fracture with minimal (<10º) extensor lag on straight leg raising
- avulsion of inferior pole of patella with intact retinaculum (as above)
- similar criteria for post–total knee patellar fracture

ALTERNATIVE TREATMENTS

- open reduction–internal fixation for displaced fractures involving the articular surface
- occasionally, open reduction–internal fixation for prosthetic patellar fractures if early during the rehabilitation course to prevent ankylosis of the total knee

SURGICAL ANATOMY

Surgical Techniques

- application of molded cylinder cast with felt above malleolae to prevent pressure sores and quadrilateral molding at thigh to enhance rotational control

POSTOPERATIVE MANAGEMENT

- typically requires 6 weeks of cast immobilization

REHABILITATION

- begin gravity-assisted passive and active range of motion at 6 weeks
- quadriceps strengthening program beginning approximately 8 weeks after injury

COMPLICATIONS

- poor cast fit and immobilization
- DVT: less of an issue with foot free; some orthopaedists use enteric-coated aspirin prophylaxis
- post-immobilization pain depends on rehabiliation

NOTES

REPAIR OF PATELLAR FRACTURE

CPT code	**27524**	**open treatment of patellar fracture, with internal fixation and/or partial or complete patellectomy and soft tissue repair**
ICD-9 codes	**822**	**fracture of patella**
	822.0	**closed**

INDICATIONS

- disruption of retinaculum with extensor lag
- >1–2-mm displacement of patellar articulating surface
- partial patellectomy for inferior pole (lower third of patella) comminution
- acute complete patellectomy only for highly comminuted, nonreconstructible fractures

ALTERNATIVE TREATMENT

- closed treatment for minimally displaced fractures with intact retinaculum

SURGICAL ANATOMY

- subcutaneous sesamoid bone
- respect the periosteum and retinaculum

APPROACHES

- use longitudinal midline or medial para-midline approach
- avoid transverse incision because of possible subsequent knee surgery

Surgical Techniques

- tension band technique: excellent long-term track record, especially for transverse fractures
  - creates compression at the fracture site
  - 2 parallel K-wires dorsal to the mid-coronal plane of the patella
  - figure-of-eight tension band, with medial and lateral twists to create symmetrical compression
- cerclage technique: use no. 5 nonresorbable suture or wire
  - may be indicated for highly comminuted fractures that will require prolonged immobilization
  - does not result in fracture compression as with tension band
- lag screw fixation: indicated only in fractures with ≥2 fracture lines to convert into compressible fracture pattern

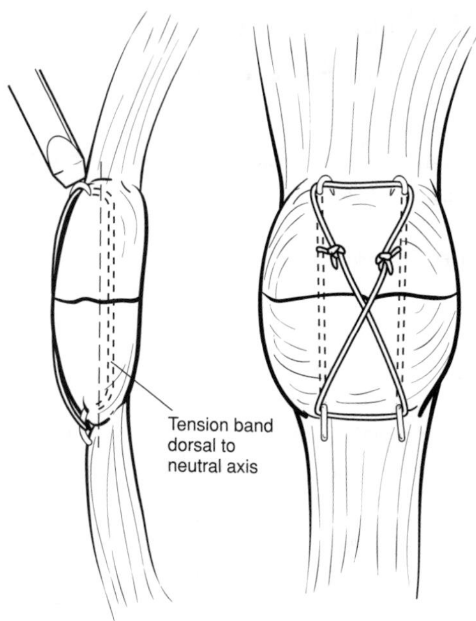

POSTOPERATIVE MANAGEMENT

- soft cast with splints for 7–10 days
- if stable construct, may begin limited flexion to 60° in polycentric locking brace
- if not stable, requires addition of cylinder cast for 6 weeks

REHABILITATION

- begin straight leg raises in cast or splint
- patient may weight-bear as tolerated
- limited flexion, even with stable construct, for 6 weeks
- if stable, allow active, gravity-assisted flexion
- avoid antigravity active extension for 6 weeks

COMPLICATIONS

- gapping at articular surface due to excessively dorsal K-wires
- tilting of articular surface and cartilage overload with distal pole recession if reattachment of patellar tendon too dorsal
- subcutaneous hardware with pain requiring removal
- late osteoarthritis

CLOSED TREATMENT OF TIBIAL PLATEAU FRACTURE

CPT code **27530 closed treatment of tibial fracture, proximal (plateau); without manipulation**

ICD-9 code **823.00 closed fracture of tibial plateau**

INDICATIONS

- minimally displaced plateau fracture
  - <2-mm displacement in young patient
  - <5-mm isolated medial or lateral displacement in ill or osteopenic patient
- mechanical (meniscal entrapment) symptoms

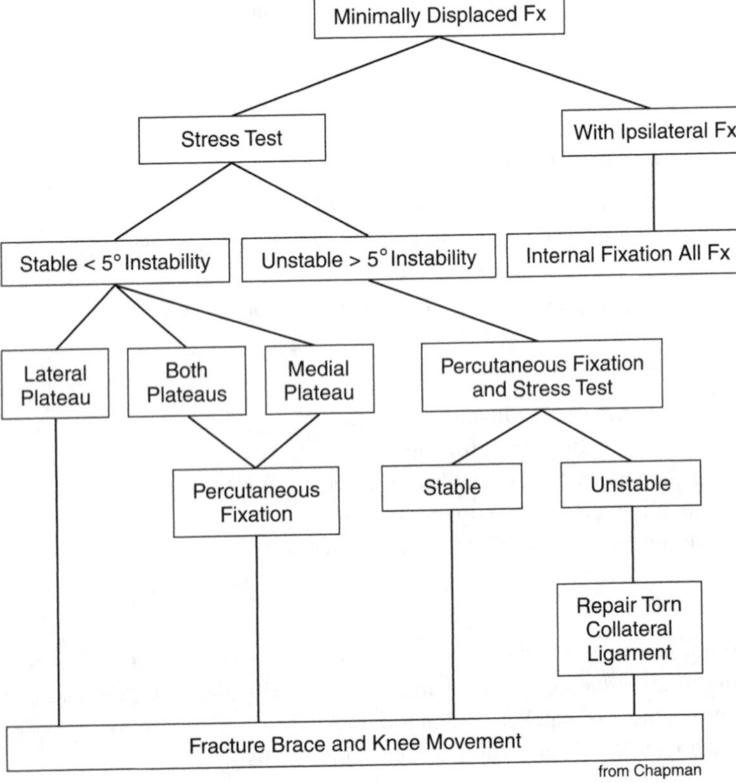

from Chapman

ALTERNATIVE TREATMENT

- open reduction–internal fixation, with elevation of depressed bone segment

APPROACHES

Surgical Techniques
- temporary application of Robert Jones or cylinder cast
- after initial decrease in swelling, consider use of a cast or Bledsoe-type brace with medial thrust pad for lateral plateau involvement

POSTOPERATIVE MANAGEMENT

- anticipate 6 weeks of immobilization

REHABILITATION

- non–weight-bearing for 6 weeks
- allow active and passive range of motion in cast or brace after 2 weeks to tolerance
- begin quadriceps and hamstring strengthening after 6 weeks
- in the elderly or infirm patient, focus on gait and balance training after healing to prevent future falls
- also, evaluation and treatment of osteoporosis beginning with immediate review of daily calcium (1500 mg) and vitamin D (50,000 U) intakes in appropriate patients

SELECTED REFERENCE

Chapman MW, Madison M (eds). Operative Orthopaedics, 2nd ed. Philadelphia: JB Lippincott, 1993.

NOTES

OPEN REDUCTION–INTERNAL FIXATION OF TIBIAL PLATEAU FRACTURE (UNICONDYLAR)

CPT code **27535 open treatment of tibial fracture, proximal (plateau); unicondylar, with or without internal or external fixation**

ICD-9 codes **823.00 tibial plateau fracture, unicondylar, closed (823.10 open)**
733.16 pathologic

INDICATIONS

- open fractures, associated compartment syndrome, vascular injury, polytrauma, displaced medial condyle fractures, and lateral condyle fractures resulting in joint instability (>10° valgus opening, >5-mm widening, >3-mm step-off).

ALTERNATIVE TREATMENTS

- cast bracing
- traction
- external fixation
- arthroscopically-assisted fixation

SURGICAL ANATOMY

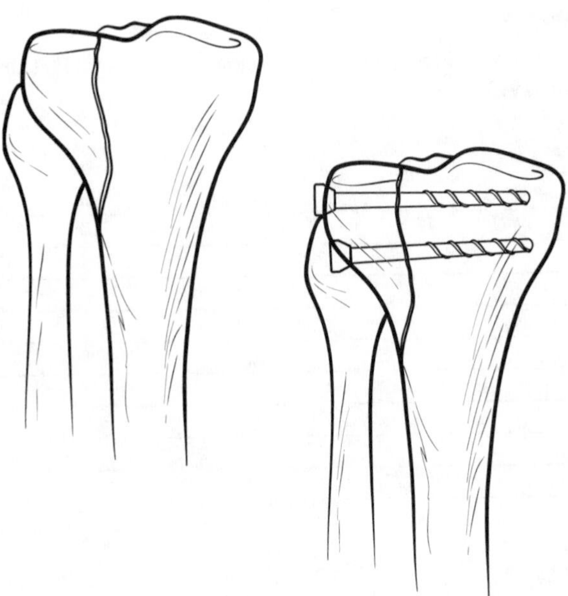

APPROACHES

- midline
- medial or lateral parapatellar

Surgical Techniques

- preoperative planning
- equipment: fluoroscope, distractor
- position: supine, bump under ipsilateral buttock
- incision: longitudinal midline, full thickness to periosteum, capsule, or fascia
- capsule divided transversely below the meniscus
- open fracture–like book cover
- joint surface reduction
- joint surface stabilization
- bone grafting as needed
- metaphyseal–diaphyseal reduction and stabilization
- mensicus repair
- final imaging
- closure

POSTOPERATIVE MANAGEMENT

- compression dressing
- elevation
- monitor for compartment syndrome

REHABILITATION

- early motion
- protected weight-bearing
- weight-bearing progressed as soon as 6–8 weeks
- full weight-bearing usually by 12–14 weeks

COMPLICATIONS

- malunion
- non-union
- infection (0–7%)
- compartment syndrome
- neurovascular injury

SELECTED REFERENCES

Honkonen SE. Indications for surgical treatment of tibial condylar fractures. Clin Orthop 1994;302:199–205.

Tscherne H, Lobenhoffer P: Tibial plateau fractures: management and expected results: a review. Clin Orthop 1993;292:87–100.

OPEN TREATMENT OF TIBIAL PLATEAU FRACTURE (BICONDYLAR)

CPT code **27536** **open treatment of tibial fracture, proximal (plateau); bicondylar, with or without internal fixation**

ICD-9 codes **823.00** **tibial plateau fracture, unicondylar, closed (823.10 open)**
733.16 **pathologic**

INDICATIONS

- all displaced closed and open fractures, associated compartment syndrome, vascular injury, polytrauma

ALTERNATIVE TREATMENTS

- cast bracing
- traction
- external fixation
- arthroscopic-assisted fixation

SURGICAL ANATOMY

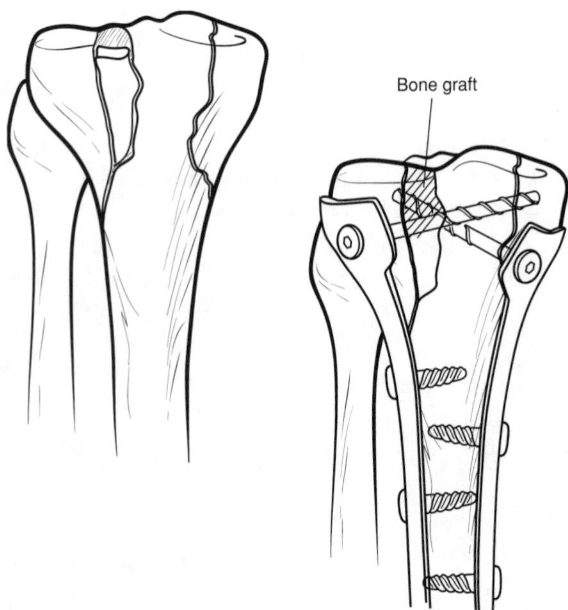

APPROACHES

- midline
- medial or lateral parapatellar
- accessory posteromedial
- patellar tendon elevation (with tubercle)

Surgical Techniques

- preoperative planning
- equipment: fluoroscope, distractor
- position: supine, bump under ipsilateral buttock
- incision: longitudinal midline, full thickness to periosteum, capsule, or fascia
- capsule divided transversely below the meniscus
- open fracture–like book cover
- joint surface reduction
- joint surface stabilization
- bone grafting as needed
- metaphyseal–diaphyseal reduction and stabilization
- mensicus repair
- final imaging
- closure

POSTOPERATIVE MANAGEMENT

- compression dressing
- elevation
- monitor for compartment syndrome

REHABILITATION

- early motion
- protected weight-bearing
- weight-bearing progressed as soon as 6–8 weeks
- full weight-bearing usually by 12–14 weeks

COMPLICATIONS

- non-union
- malunion
- infection (0–7%)
- compartment syndrome
- neurovascular injury

SELECTED REFERENCES

Honkonen SE. Indications for surgical treatment of tibial condylar fractures. Clin Orthop 1994;302:199–205.

Tscherne H, Lobenhoffer P. Tibial plateau fractures: management and expected results: a review. Clin Orthop 1993;292:87–100.

NOTES

CLOSED REDUCTION OF KNEE DISLOCATION

CPT code	**27550 closed treatment of knee dislocation, without anesthesia**
ICD-9 codes	**836.50 dislocation of knee, closed, unspecified**
	836.50–836.59 other dislocations of knee, closed

INDICATIONS

- any knee dislocation in any plane that is reducible
- documentation of neurovascular status is mandatory

ALTERNATIVE TREATMENTS

- closed reduction under general anesthesia
- open reduction

ANATOMY

- determine neurovascular status
- determine direction of dislocation: anterior, posterior, medial, lateral, or rotational

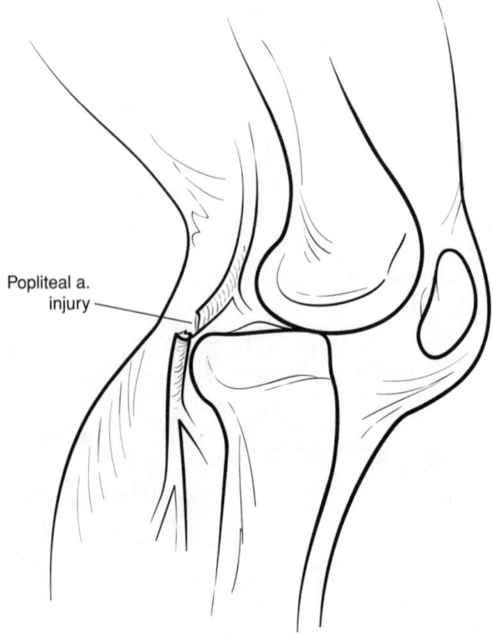

- determine structures damaged
- most authors recommend arteriograms; presence of pulse does not exclude intimal injury

APPROACHES

Manipulation Techniques

- anterior: traction plus elevation of distal femur
- posterior: traction plus extension and lifting of proximal anterior tibia
- medial and lateral: traction plus appropriate translation of femur and tibia
- rotational: traction plus appropriate derotation of tibia
- concurrent ligament repair is controversial

POSTOPERATIVE MANAGEMENT

- document neurologic and vascular status before and after any attempt at reduction
- knee immobilized in 20–30º of flexion until further evaluation
- do not apply circular plaster cast or constricting dressing

REHABILITATION

- elevation
- mobilize foot and ankle
- non–weight-bearing ambulation

COMPLICATIONS

- vascular: popliteal artery 25–30% of all dislocations
- neurologic: peroneal nerve 14–35%
- ligamentous: cruciates, collaterals
- irreducible: posterolateral dislocation: "dimple sign" on medial joint line requires emergent reduction under general anesthesia

SELECTED REFERENCES

Cole BJ, Harner CD. The multiple ligament injured knee. Clin Sports Med 1999;18(1): 241–262.

Miranda FE, Dennis JW, Veldenz HC, et al. Confirmation of the safety and accuracy of physical examination in the evaluation of knee dislocation for injury of the popliteal artery: a prospective study. J Trauma 2002;52(2):247–251.

CLOSED REDUCTION OF PATELLAR DISLOCATION

CPT code **27560 closed treatment of patellar dislocation, without anesthesia**

ICD-9 code **836.3 dislocation of knee, dislocation of patella, closed**

INDICATION

- patella dislocation in a cooperative patient

ALTERNATIVE TREATMENTS

- closed reduction with local anesthesia
- closed reduction under general anesthesia
- open treatment for displaced intra-articular fractures
- open reduction of intra-articular dislocations

APPROACHES

Manipulation Techniques

- arthrocentesis to decompress knee and look for fat globules to rule out osteochondral fracture
- extension and gentle manipulation of the patella

POSTOPERATIVE MANAGEMENT

- controversial
- cast or brace in extension for ambulation for 3 weeks

REHABILITATION

- quadriceps setting exercises
- straight leg raises with and without weights
- short and long arc quadriceps exercises with and without weights
- range of motion

COMPLICATIONS

- osteochondral fractures of the medial edge of the patella, 5%

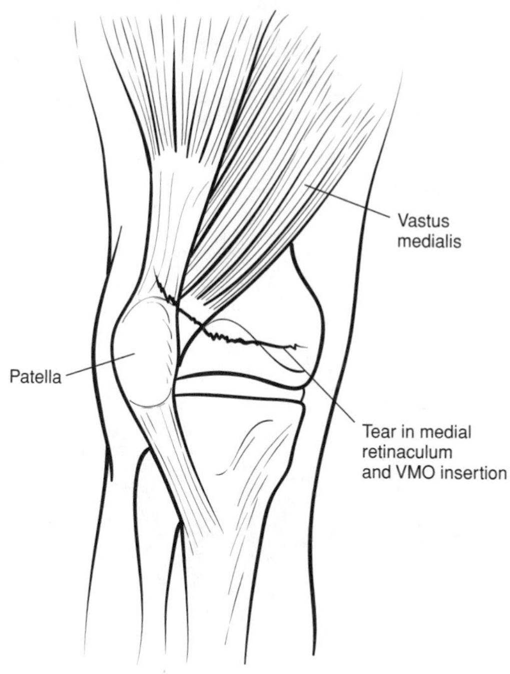
Vastus
medialis
Patella
Tear in medial
retinaculum
and VMO insertion

NOTES

PART VIII

CALF & ANKLE

DECOMPRESSIVE FASCIOTOMY, CALF

CPT code	**27602**	**decompression fasciotomy, leg, anterior and/or lateral, and posterior compartment(s)**
ICD-9 codes	**958.8**	**other early complications of trauma**
	906	**late effects of injuries to skin and subcutaneous tissues**
	906.4	**late effect of crushing**

INDICATIONS

- compartment syndrome is a clinical diagnosis
- remember the 6 "Ps": pain, pressure, pain with passive stretch, paresis, paresthesias, and pulses
- confirmation by compartment pressures
  - >30–35 mm Hg
  - within 30 mm Hg of diastolic blood pressure

ALTERNATIVE TREATMENT

- none; the only accepted treatment for acute compartment syndrome is fasciotomy (see CPT 20950, compartment pressure measurement p. 40)

SURGICAL ANATOMY

Incision

- 2 vertical skin incisions (with >8 cm skin bridge)
- lateral incision over the interval between anterior and lateral compartments
- medial incision 2 cm behind the posterolateral border tibia

APPROACHES

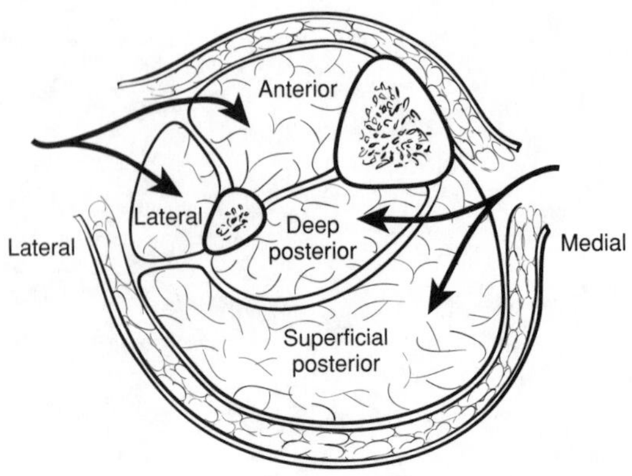

Surgical Techniques

- lateral
  - identify superficial peroneal nerve
  - release anterior compartment 1 cm anterior to septum
  - release lateral compartment 1 cm posterior to septum
- medial
  - identify saphenous vein and nerve
  - release fascia over gastrocnemius soleus (superficial post compartment)
  - release fascia over deep post compartment (detach part of soleal bridge)
  - pack wounds open

POSTOPERATIVE MANAGEMENT

- return to operating room every 36–72 hours for dressing change; gradual wound closure
- split thickness skin graft at 7–10 days if wounds cannot be closed primarily

REHABILITATION

- weight-bearing status depends on associated injuries

COMPLICATIONS

- inadequate compartment release (ischemic contracture)
- nerve damage (superficial peroneal, saphenous)

SELECTED REFERENCE

Amendola A, Twaddle BC. Compartment syndrome. In: Browner BD, et al, eds. Skeletal trauma. Philadelphia: WB Saunders, 1998:365–389.

NOTES

PERCUTANEOUS ACHILLES TENOTOMY

CPT code **27606 tenotomy, percutaneous, Achilles tendon (separate procedure); general anesthesia**

ICD-9 code **727.81 short Achilles tendon (acquired)**

INDICATION

- significant Achilles tendon contracture with symptomatic, associated foot or ankle symptoms or gait disturbance nonresponsive to conservative treatment

ALTERNATIVE TREATMENTS

- Achilles tendon stretching, heel lift
- open Z-lengthening of Achilles tendon
- gastrocnemius recession (preferable if ankle dorsiflexion is restricted with knee extension but not with knee flexion)

SURGICAL ANATOMY

- Achilles tendon is common at the insertion of the gastrocnemius and soleus muscles on the calcaneus; the tendon fibers internally rotate approximately 90° as they course distally

Incision

- 2 or 3 transverse incisions over Achilles tendon

APPROACHES

Surgical Techniques

- Hoke's technique
  - percutaneously cut medial 50% of tendon 2 and 7 cm from the calcaneal insertion with no. 15 or no. 11 blade
  - cut lateral 50% of tendon about 4.5 cm from insertion
- White's technique
  - percutaneously cut anterior 50% of tendon 2 cm from the calcaneal insertion
  - cut medial 50% of tendon 7 cm from the calcaneal insertion
- both: passively dorsiflex foot elongating tendon

POSTOPERATIVE MANAGEMENT

- cast immobilization for 6 weeks

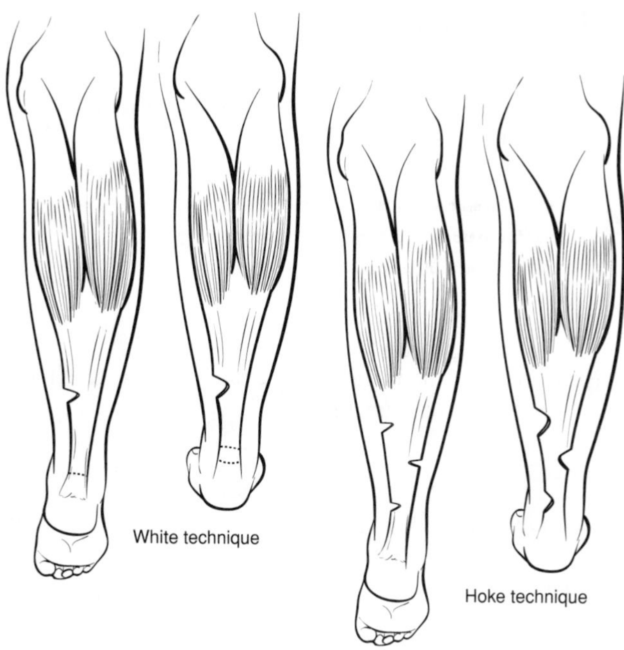

REHABILITATION

- TDWB in cast, then WBAT in cam walker for 2–6 weeks
- physical therapy for stretching and strengthening Achilles tendon

COMPLICATIONS

- weakness (Achilles tendon overlengthening)
- intraoperative tendon rupture (heals in cast)
- Achilles tendinitis

SELECTED REFERENCES

Hoke M. An operation for the correction of extremely relaxed flat feet. J Bone Joint Surg 1931;13:773–783.

White JC. Torsion of the achilles tendon: its surgical significance. Arch Surg 1943; 46:784–787.

NOTES

ARTHROTOMY, ANKLE

CPT code	**27610 arthrotomy, ankle, including exploration, drainage, or removal of foreign body**
ICD-9 codes	**711.07 pyogenic arthritis of foot and ankle**
	718.17 loose body in joint of foot and ankle
	726.91 exostosis of unspecified site

INDICATION

- symptomatic ankle loose body, infection, exostosis, or osteochondral lesion not amenable to arthroscopic treatment

ALTERNATIVE TREATMENT

- ankle arthroscopy

SURGICAL ANATOMY

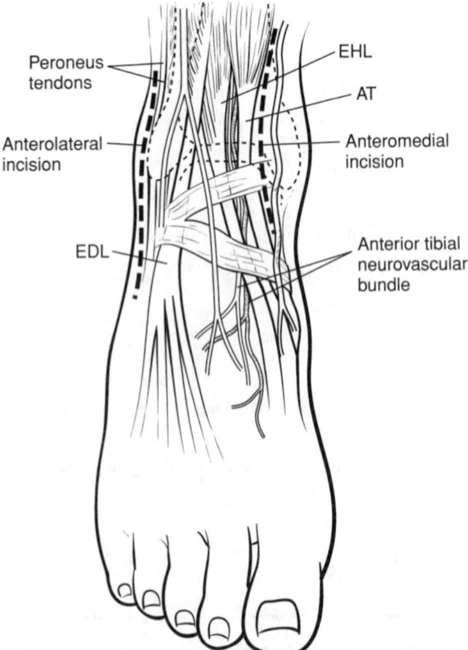

Incision

- anteromedial: medial to anterior tibial tendon
- anterolateral: lateral to peroneus tertius tendon
- posterolateral: between Achilles and peroneal tendons
- posteromedial: between Achilles and flexor hallucis longus tendons

APPROACHES

Surgical Techniques

- position: supine
- incision: anteromedial or anterolateral most common
- protect nerves
  - anteromedial: saphenous
  - anterolateral: superficial peroneal
  - posterolateral: sural
  - posteromedial: tibial
- address pathology
- close capsule and skin

POSTOPERATIVE MANAGEMENT

- compressive dressing and posterior splint

REHABILITATION

- WBAT in cam walker at 4–7 days
- ankle range of motion and strengthening exercises

COMPLICATIONS

- neurologic injury
- infection
- wound dehiscence
- synovial fistula

NOTES

EXCISION GANGLION CYST, ANKLE

CPT code **27630** **excision of lesion of tendon sheath or capsule (e.g., cyst or ganglion), leg and/or ankle**

ICD-9 codes **727.40** **synovial cyst, unspecified**
727.41 **ganglion of joint**
727.42 **ganglion of tendon sheath**

INDICATION

- mass that is symptomatic or possibly malignant

ALTERNATIVE TREATMENTS

- benign neglect if asymptomatic
- decrease pressure on mass (donut pads, soft leather shoes, skipping shoelace holes over mass)
- aspiration with or without cortisone injection

SURGICAL ANATOMY

Incision

- longitudinal extensile incision over mass

APPROACHES

Surgical Techniques

- longitudinal extensile incision over mass
- stay in 1 anatomic compartment
- protect neurovascular structures
- excise entire mass and send for pathology
- excise stalk of ganglion and repair rent in capsule
- close skin

POSTOPERATIVE MANAGEMENT

- compressive dressing with or without splint, brace, or surgical shoe

REHABILITATION

- WBAT
- range of motion and strengthening exercises

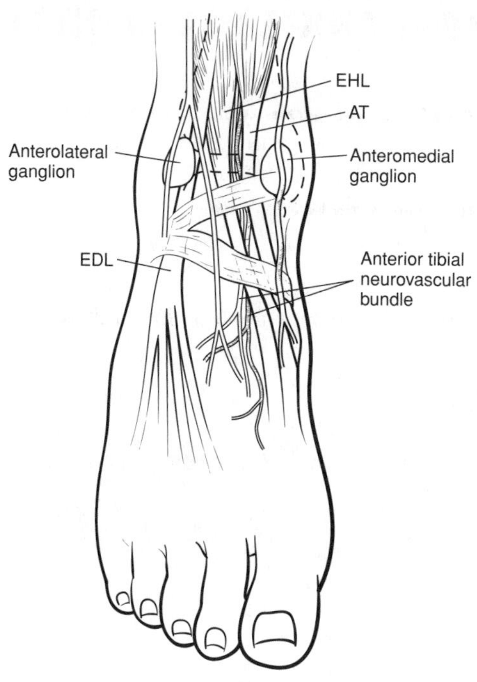

COMPLICATIONS

- recurrence
- infection
- neurologic injury
- wound dehiscence

NOTES

DEBRIDEMENT ANKLE OSTEOPHYTE

CPT code **27640** **partial excision (craterization, saucerization, or diaphysectomy), bone (e.g., osteomyelitis or exostosis); tibia**

ICD-9 code **726.91** **exostosis, any bone (specify)**

INDICATION

- spurring of anterior tibia blocking dorsiflexion of the ankle

SURGICAL ANATOMY

Incision

- anterolateral approach to the ankle and then subperiosteal dissection across the anterior tibia

APPROACHES

Surgical Techniques

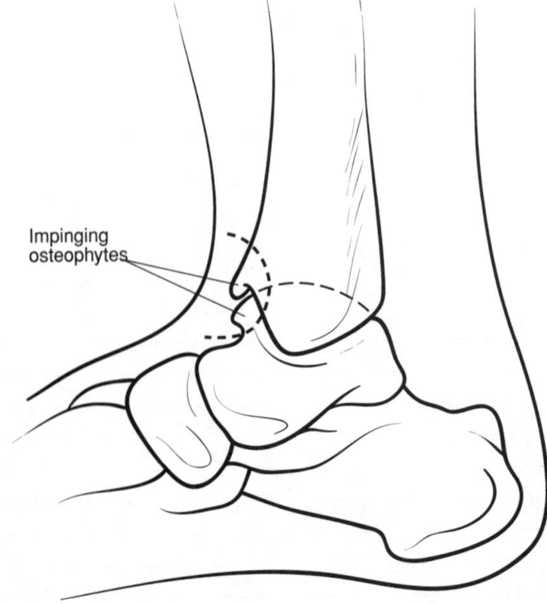

- use osteotome across anterior tibia and "angle" the osteotome so as to remove the spur and a few millimeters of normal tibia; this helps avoid recurrence of the spur
- consider lengthening the Achilles tendon if dorsiflexion is not adequate after tibial resection

POSTOPERATIVE MANAGEMENT

- if surgical lengthening of Achilles tendon is performed, nonweight bearing cast in neutral dorsiflexion for 8 weeks, and then mobilize
- if lengthening of the Achilles tendon is not performed, hold in neutral dorsiflexion for 2–4 weeks and then mobilize

COMPLICATIONS

- be careful, when moving the osteotome from lateral to medial, not to fracture the medial malleolus
- care must be taken to not take too much of the anterior joint with the resection

SELECTED REFERENCE

Hansen ST. Functional reconstruction of the foot and ankle. Philadelphia: Lippincott, 2000.

NOTES

REPAIR OF ACHILLES TENDON RUPTURE

CPT code **27650 repair, primary, open or percutaneous, ruptured Achilles tendon**

ICD-9 codes **845.09 Achilles tendon rupture, traumatic**
727.67 Achilles tendon rupture, nontraumatic

INDICATION

- Achilles tendon rupture in adult

ALTERNATIVE TREATMENT

- casting in equinus in patient who is elderly or not a surgical candidate

SURGICAL ANATOMY

Incision
- posterolateral: along lateral border of Achilles tendon
- some surgeons use posteromedial

APPROACHES

Surgical Techniques
- position: prone or "sloppy" lateral with a bean bag
- incision: along lateral border of Achilles tendon
- stay on anterior border of Achilles tendon; do not separate tendon from overlying skin
- repair with no. 2 or 5 Ticron or similar suture (modified Kessler or Krackow—see p. 181)
- consider FHL or peroneus brevis tendon transfer if the defect is major or difficult to reapproximate

POSTOPERATIVE MANAGEMENT

- usually outpatient or 1 day in hospital
- physical therapy for crutch-walking or non–weight-bearing on operative extremity

REHABILITATION

- non–weight-bearing for 6 weeks (some surgeons begin WBAT in cam walker at 2–3 weeks)
- cast in gravity equinus for 3 weeks and then cast at neutral dorsiflexion for 3 weeks
- begin weight-bearing at 8 weeks with 0.25-in. heel lift added to sole of shoe

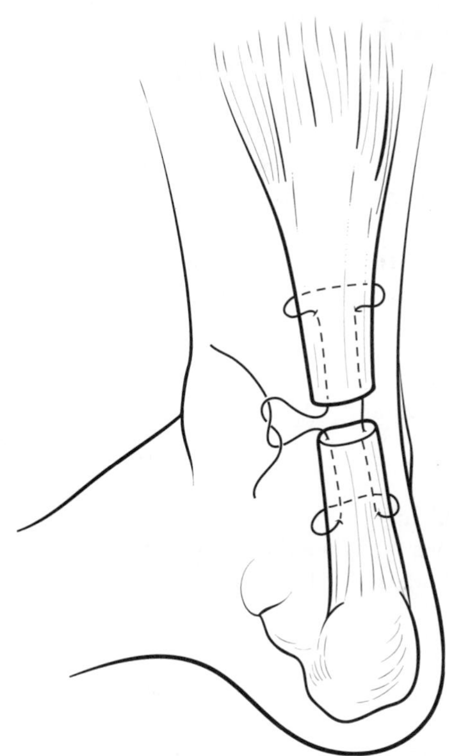

- remove lift after 1 month of weight-bearing
- formal therapy if required

COMPLICATIONS

- rerupture <1%
- skin necrosis: greater if incision too posterior or skin is separated from underlying tendon

NOTES

CLOSED TREATMENT OF TIBIAL SHAFT FRACTURE

CPT code **27750 closed treatment of tibial shaft fracture (with or without fibular fracture), without manipulation**

ICD-9 codes **823.20 closed fracture of shaft of tibia**
823.22 closed fracture of shaft of fibula with tibia

INDICATION

- nondisplaced, low-energy fracture

ALTERNATIVE TREATMENTS

- intramedullary rodding
- open reduction–internal fixation with plate
- external fixator if grade II or III open fracture

ANATOMY

- rule out compartment syndrome before applying circumferential cast or dressing
- peroneal nerve is subcutaneous approximately 3 cm below fibular head

APPROACHES

- proximal or midshaft fractures require long leg cast for 6 weeks
- low-energy distal third fractures may be treated in a well-molded short leg or patellar tendon-bearing cast if fibula is intact

MANAGEMENT

- if fracture is entirely stable, it can be monitored by x-ray in 1–2 weeks
- if fracture is initially angulated, it requires follow-up x-ray in 3–5 days and then weekly for several weeks
- proximal fracture treated in long leg cast requires 6 weeks of immobilization and usually an additional 4–6 weeks of short leg casting thereafter
- proximal or distal metaphyseal fractures will heal to tolerate weight-bearing in 6–8 weeks
- average time to healing for middle or distal third diaphyseal fracture is 16–20 weeks
- role of cast bracing is controversial

REHABILITATION

- initial toe-touch weight-bearing; depending on the fracture, progress depends on location, tenderness, and x-ray appearance
- consider knee range of motion as soon as allowed by short leg cast

COMPLICATIONS

- delayed healing or progressive varus deformity with intact fibula
- knee or ankle stiffness postimmobilization
- muscle atrophy secondary to limited function
- disuse osteoporosis of tibia and adjacent bones

NOTES

PLATING TIBIAL SHAFT FRACTURE

CPT code **27758 open treatment of tibial shaft fracture (with or without fibular fracture) with plate/screws**

ICD-9 codes **823.20 closed fracture of shaft of tibia**
823.22 closed fracture of shaft of fibula with tibia

INDICATION

- low-energy closed fracture of diaphysis

ALTERNATIVE TREATMENTS

- closed treatment for stable fracture configurations
- intramedullary rodding
- external fixator for open grade II or III fractures

SURGICAL ANATOMY

- tibia is subcutaneous throughout the diaphysis
- protect patellar tendon insertion proximally
- avoid plunging with drills or taps in sagittal plane, especially at trifurcation (1 hand breadth below joint line)
- avoid deep and superficial peroneal branches distally above ankle joint line

Incision

- depends on location of fracture

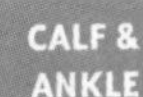

Surgical Techniques

- longitudinal incision lateral to tibial crest
- use lateral surface for tibial plating to avoid subcutaneous hardware
- minimum of 8 cortices of fixation proximal and distal to fracture
- specialized plates are available for proximal or distal fractures that propagate into the diaphyseal region

POSTOPERATIVE MANAGEMENT

- soft, dry sterile dressing if fixation is stable
- routine DVT prophylaxis with enteric coated aspirin at a minimum
- immediately begin knee and ankle range of motion
- weight-bearing depends on fracture configuration

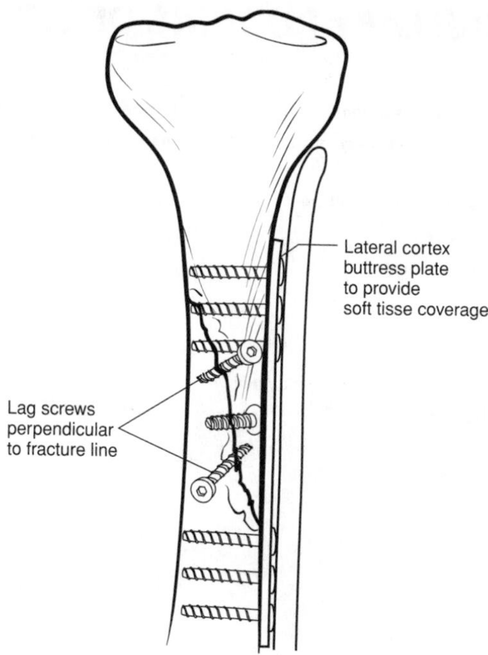

REHABILITATION

- typically will require limited weight-bearing for at least 8 weeks postoperatively
- begin knee and ankle range of motion; include subtalar range of motion home exercise program
- with clinical and radiographic healing, progress weight-bearing and begin BAPS foot and ankle mobilization

COMPLICATIONS

- infection: recognize that, with open fractures, staging depends on soft tissues and not solely on size of laceration
- delayed healing, particularly in distal third diaphysis
- late hardware bursitis if prominent
- plate-associated osteoporosis secondary to stress shielding

NOTES

INTRAMEDULLARY RODDING OF TIBIA

CPT code **27759** **open treatment of tibial shaft fracture (with or without fibular fracture) by intramedullary implant, with or without interlocking screws and/or cerclage**

ICD-9 codes **823.20** **tibia shaft fracture**
823.30 **open**
733.16 **pathologic**

INDICATION

- tibial diaphyseal open fractures, compartment syndrome, arterial injury, polytrauma, "floating knee," or fractures that cannot be stabilized by closed means

ALTERNATIVE TREATMENTS

- cast
- fracture brace
- plate fixation
- external fixation

SURGICAL ANATOMY

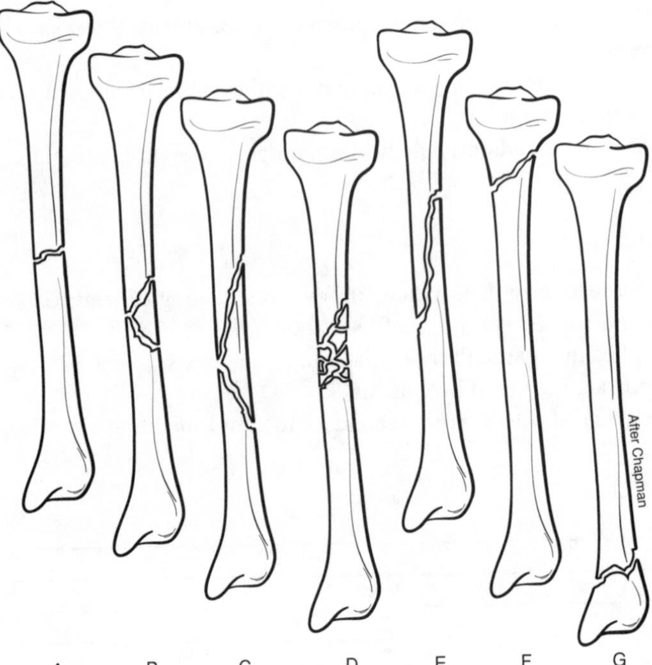

APPROACH

- medial parapatellar

Surgical Techniques

- preoperative planning
- equipment: fracture table or distractor, fluoroscope
- position: supine
- incision: medial parapatellar incision
- patellar tendon retracted laterally
- central starting point viewed on fluoroscope
- proximal tibia opened
- fracture reduced
- ball tip guidewire inserted
- tibia reamed
- nail size determined
- guidewire exchanged for smooth tip
- nail inserted
- fracture distraction eliminated
- transverse locking screws placed
- final imaging
- closure

POSTOPERATIVE MANAGEMENT

- compression dressing
- elevation
- monitor for compartment syndrome

REHABILITATION

- early motion
- protected weight-bearing
- weight-bearing progressed as soon as 6–8 wks (earlier if transverse)
- full weight-bearing usually by 12–14 wks

COMPLICATIONS

- knee stiffness
- infection
- delayed or non-union
- malunion
- hardware failure
- compartment syndrome
- neurovascular injury

SELECTED REFERENCES

Bone LB, Johnson KD. Treatment of tibial fractures by reaming and intramedullary nailing. J Bone Joint Surg 1986;68A:877–887.

Singer RW, Kellam JF. Open tibial diaphyseal fractures: results of unreamed locked intramedullary nailing. Clin Orthop 1995;315:114–118.

NOTES

OPEN REDUCTION–INTERNAL FIXATION OF MEDIAL MALLEOLUS

CPT code **27766 open treatment of medial malleolus fracture, with or without internal or external fixation**

ICD-9 codes **824.0 (closed fracture)**
824.1 (open fracture)

INDICATIONS

- open fracture
- nonanatomic reduction after closed manipulaiton
- after successful closed reduction, when the foot must be maintained in an extreme position to hold the reduction or with a very unstable fracture

ALTERNATIVE TREATMENT

- closed reduction and casting with closed stable fracture; anatomic reduction after manipulation

SURGICAL ANATOMY

Incision

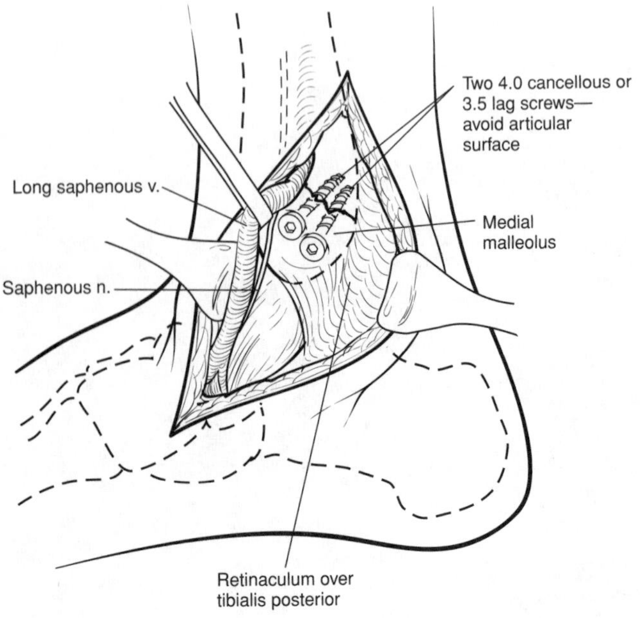

APPROACHES

Surgical Techniques

- supine position
- thigh tourniquet
- medial incision (usually 5–8 cm)
- avoid injury to saphenous nerve and vein
- anatomic reduction of fracture
- internal fixation with screws; consider external fixation with open fracture
- atraumatic wound closure

POSTOPERATIVE MANAGEMENT

- short leg compressive dressing with splint for 1–2 weeks, ankle neutral
- hinged ankle brace or cam walker for subsequent 4 weeks (toe touch weight-bearing)
- progress to full weight-bearing in brace at 6 weeks postoperatively

REHABILITATION

- active range of motion and gentle ankle passive range of motion in hinged ankle brace
- aggressive active and passive range of motion, strengthening, and agility exercises begin 6 weeks postoperatively

COMPLICATIONS

- neurovascular injury
- loss of reduction, particularly with osteopenic bone
- osteoarthritis secondary to cartilage injury or inadequate reduction
- infection

SELECTED REFERENCES

Carr JB, Trafton PG. Malleolar fractures and soft tissue injuries of the ankle. In: Browner BD, Jupiter JB, Levine AM, Trafton PG, eds. Skeletal trauma, 2nd ed. Philadelphia: WB Saunders, 1998.

Wilson FC. The pathogenesis and treatment of ankle fractures: classification. Instruct Course Lect 1990;39:79–83.

Wilson FC. The pathogenesis and treatment of ankle fractures: historical studies. Instruct Course Lect 1990;39:73–78.

NOTES

CLOSED TREATMENT OF LATERAL MALLEOLAR FRACTURE

CPT code **27786** **closed treatment of distal fibular fracture (lateral malleolus), without manipulation**

ICD-9 code **824.2** **closed fracture of distal fibula (lateral malleolus)**

INDICATIONS

- nondisplaced fracture

ALTERNATIVE TREATMENT

- open reduction–internal fixation

Manipulation Technique

- if nondisplaced, cast *in situ*
- if displaced, reduce/cast in inversion/internal rotation
- if nondisplaced, short leg walking cast with foot and ankle in neutral position for 2 weeks; *then*
- if displaced, short leg nonweightbearing cast for 4 weeks; *then*
- hinged ankle brace, full weight-bearing for total of 6 weeks

REHABILITATION

- begin aggressive ankle passive and active range of motion at 4 weeks
- strengthening and agility exercises begin 6 weeks postoperatively

COMPLICATIONS

- loss of reduction
- missed syndesmotic injury
- late osteoarthritis

SELECTED REFERENCES

Carr JB, Trafton PG. Malleolar fractures and soft tissue injuries of the ankle. In: Browner BD, Jupiter JB, Levine AM, Trafton PG, eds. Skeletal trauma, 2nd ed. Philadelphia: WB Saunders, 1998.

Wilson FC. The pathogenesis and treatment of ankle fractures: classification. Instruct Course Lect 1990;39:79–83.

Wilson FC. The pathogenesis and treatment of ankle fractures: historical studies. Instruct Course Lect 1990;39:73–78.

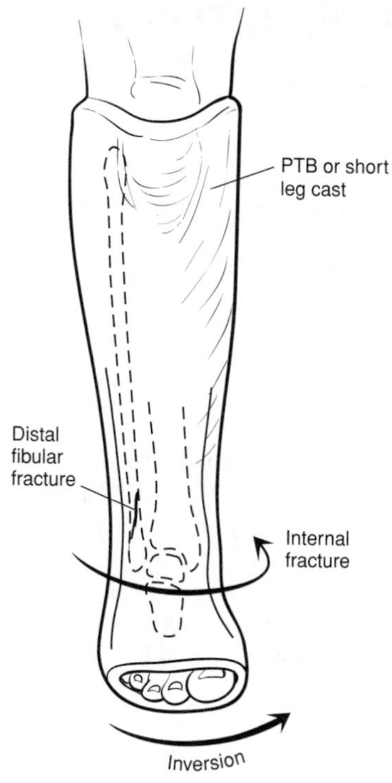
PTB or short leg cast
Distal fibular fracture
Internal fracture
Inversion

NOTES

OPEN REDUCTION–INTERNAL FIXATION OF LATERAL MALLEOLUS

CPT code	**27792**	**open treatment of distal fibular fracture (lateral malleolus), with or without internal or external fixation**
ICD-9 codes	**824.2**	**closed fracture**
	824.3	**open fracture**

INDICATIONS

- open fracture
- nonanatomic reduction after closed manipulation
- after successful closed reduction, when the foot must be maintained in an extreme position to hold the reduction, or with a very unstable fracture

ALTERNATIVE TREATMENT

- closed reduction and casting with closed stable fracture; anatomic reduction after manipulation

APPROACH

- lateral

SURGICAL ANATOMY

Surgical Techniques

- supine position
- thigh tourniquet
- lateral incision
- avoid injury to sural and superficial peroneal nerves
- anatomic reduction of fracture
- internal fixation with screws; consider external fixation with open fracture
- usually add ⅓ tubular buttress plate (not illustrated)
- atraumatic wound closure

POSTOPERATIVE MANAGEMENT

- short leg compressive dressing with splint for 1–2 weeks, with ankle neutral
- hinged ankle brace for subsequent 4 weeks
- progress to full weight-bearing in brace at 6 weeks postoperatively

Incision

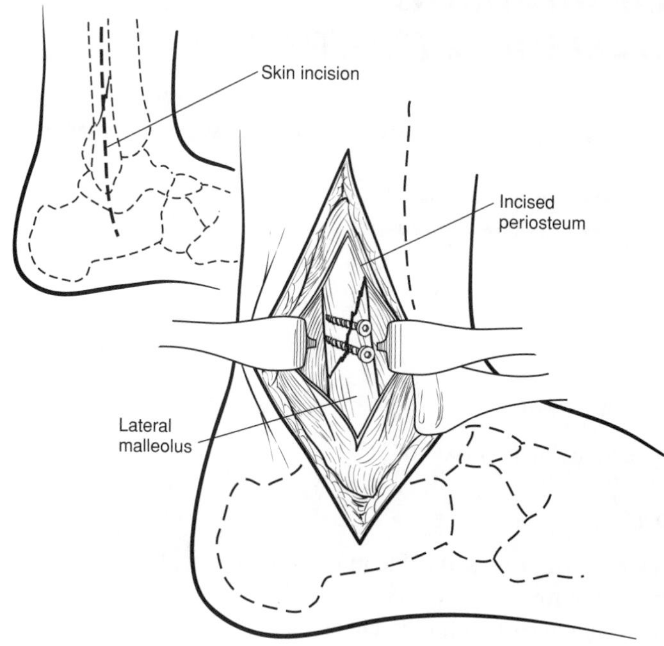

REHABILITATION

- active range of motion and gentle ankle passive range of motion in hinged ankle brace
- aggressive active and passive range of motion, strengthening, and agility exercises begin 6 weeks postoperatively

COMPLICATIONS

- neurovascular injury
- loss of reduction, particularly with osteopenic bone
- osteoarthritis secondary to cartilage injury or inadequate reduction
- infection

SELECTED REFERENCES

Carr JB, Trafton PG. Malleolar fractures and soft tissue injuries of the ankle. In: Browner BD, Jupiter JB, Levine AM, Trafton PG, eds. Skeletal trauma, 2nd ed. Philadelphia: WB Saunders, 1998.

Wilson FC. The pathogenesis and treatment of ankle fractures: classification. Instruct Course Lect 1990;39:79–83.

Wilson FC. The pathogenesis and treatment of ankle fractures: historical studies. Instruct Course Lect 1990;39:73–78.

CLOSED TREATMENT OF BIMALLEOLAR FRACTURE

CPT code **27808 closed treatment of bimalleolar ankle fracture, without manipulation**

ICD-9 codes **824 fracture of ankle**
824.4 bimalleolar, closed

INDICATION

- nondisplaced fracture

ALTERNATIVE TREATMENT

- open reduction–internal fixation

MANAGEMENT

- short leg cast with foot and ankle in neutral position; touch-down weight-bearing for 2 weeks; *then*
- short leg walking cast with foot and ankle in neutral position, partial weight-bearing for 2 weeks; *then*
- hinged ankle brace with full weight-bearing for 2 weeks

REHABILITATION

- begin ankle passive and active range of motion at 4 weeks
- strengthening and agility exercises begin 6 weeks postoperatively

COMPLICATIONS

- loss of reduction
- soft tissue necrosis with poor cast technique

SELECTED REFERENCES

Carr JB, Trafton PG. Malleolar fractures and soft tissue injuries of the ankle. In: Browner BD, Jupiter JB, Levine AM, Trafton PG, eds. Skeletal trauma, 2nd ed. Philadelphia: WB Saunders, 1998.

Wilson FC. The pathogenesis and treatment of ankle fractures: classification. Instruct Course Lect 1990;39:79–83.

Wilson FC. The pathogenesis and treatment of ankle fractures: historical studies. Instruct Course Lect 1990;39:73–78.

NOTES

OPEN REDUCTION–INTERNAL FIXATION OF BIMALLEOLAR FRACTURE

CPT code	**27814**	**open treatment of bimalleolar ankle fracture, with or without internal or external fixation**
ICD-9 codes	**824.4**	**closed**
	824.5	**open**

INDICATIONS

- open fracture
- nonanatomic reduction after closed manipulation
- after successful closed reduction, when the foot must be maintained in an extreme position to hold the reduction, or with a very unstable fracture

ALTERNATIVE TREATMENT

- closed reduction and casting with closed stable fracture; anatomic reduction after manipulation

APPROACHES

- medial approach for medial malleolus (see CPT 27766)
- lateral approach for lateral malleolus (see CPT 27792)

SURGICAL ANATOMY

Surgical Techniques

- supine position
- thigh tourniquet
- medial incision
  - avoid injury to saphenous nerve and vein
- lateral incision
  - avoid injury to sural and superficial peroneal nerves
- anatomic reduction of fractures
- internal fixation with plate and screws laterally and screw(s) medially; consider external fixation with open fracture
- atraumatic wound closure

POSTOPERATIVE MANAGEMENT

- short leg compressive dressing with splint for 1–2 weeks, ankle neutral
- hinged ankle brace for subsequent 4 weeks
- progress to full weight-bearing in brace at 6 weeks postoperatively

REHABILITATION

- active range of motion and gentle ankle passive range of motion in hinged ankle brace
- aggressive active and passive range of motion, strengthening, and agility exercises begin 6 weeks postoperatively

COMPLICATIONS

- neurovascular injury
- loss of reduction, particularly with osteopenic bone
- osteoarthritis secondary to cartilage injury or inadequate reduction
- infection

SELECTED REFERENCES

Carr JB, Trafton PG. Malleolar fractures and soft tissue injuries of the ankle. In: Browner BD, Jupiter JB, Levine AM, Trafton PG, eds. Skeletal trauma, 2nd ed. Philadelphia: WB Saunders, 1998.

Wilson FC. The pathogenesis and treatment of ankle fractures: classification. Instruct Course Lect 1990;39:79–83.

Wilson FC. The pathogenesis and treatment of ankle fractures: historical studies. Instruct Course Lect 1990;39:73–78.

NOTES

CLOSED TREATMENT OF ANKLE DISLOCATION

CPT code **27842 closed treatment of ankle dislocation; requiring anesthesia, with or without percutaneous skeletal fixation**

ICD-9 codes **837.0 closed**
837.1 open

INDICATION

- closed ankle dislocation

SURGICAL TECHNIQUES

- reduce with traction, reversal of deformity
- rarely requires percutaneous fixation to maintain reduction

POSTOPERATIVE MANAGEMENT

- short leg cast, non–weight-bearing for 6 weeks, *then*
- ambulation in a hinged brace for 2 weeks
- remove percutaneous fixation, if used, at 4–6 weeks

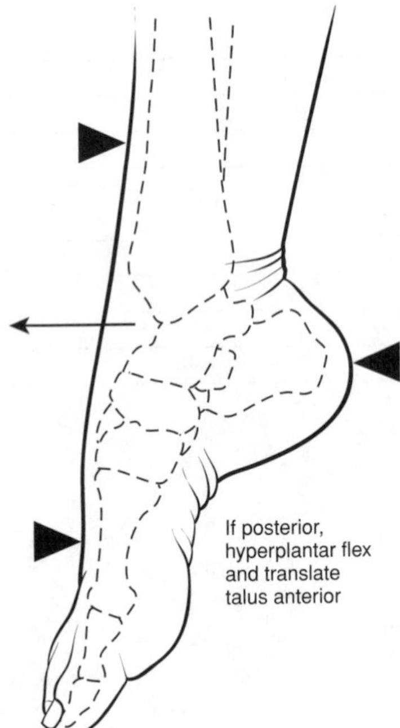

REHABILITATION

- aggressive active and passive range of motion and strengthening begin at 6 weeks

COMPLICATIONS

- neurovascular injury
- ligamentous instability

NOTES

ANKLE ARTHRODESIS

CPT code **27870 arthrodesis, ankle, any method**

ICD-9 code **715.17 osteoarthrosis, localized, primary, involving ankle and foot**

INDICATIONS

- arthritis: posttraumatic, rheumatoid, degenerative
- infection
- postpoliomyelitis weakness
- severe deformity
- avascular necrosis of talus
- salvage of failed total ankle replacement

ALTERNATIVE TREATMENTS

- bracing
- total ankle arthroplasty

SURGICAL ANATOMY (SEE ALSO CPT 27610, p. 210)

Incision

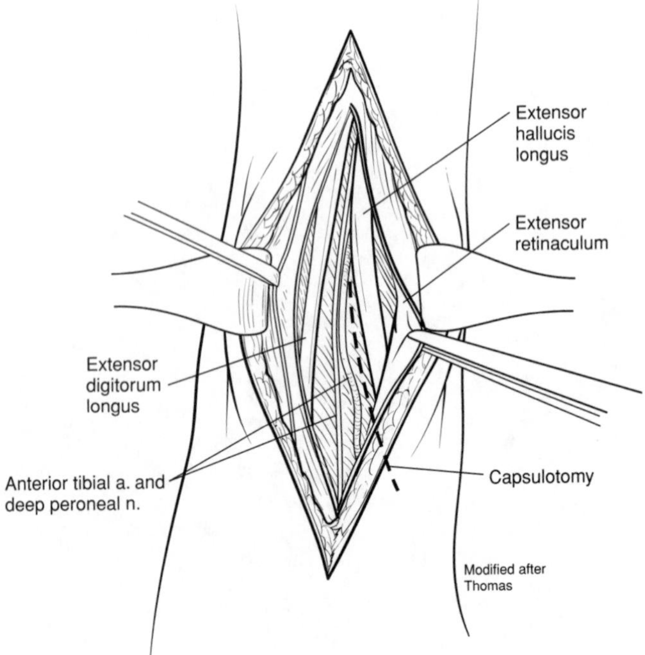

APPROACHES

- medial and lateral transmalleolar approach with lateral fixation
- anteromedial or anterolateral approach with sliding tibia graft and anterior fixation
- posterior approach with posterior grafting and fixation
- arthroscopic arthrodesis with percutaneous fixation
- any of the above with external fixation compressive arthrodesis

Surgical Techniques

- medial and lateral transmalleolar approach with lateral fixation
  - supine position
  - thigh tourniquet
  - medial incision and medial malleolar osteotomy (as needed)
  - lateral incision, distal fibular osteotomy, and partial excision of distal fibula
  - cartilage removal and creation of congruent opposing subchondral surfaces
  - internal fixation with compression screws or plate across medial malleolus and lateral blade plate
  - optimum position of internal fixation: neutral plantar flexion and dorsiflexion, 5–10° external rotation, 0–5° hindfoot valgus
  - use resected fibula as bone graft

POSTOPERATIVE MANAGEMENT

- short leg cast, non–weight-bearing for 6–10 weeks
- short leg walking cast, full weight-bearing for 4–6 weeks

REHABILITATION

- gait training
- rocker-bottom shoe

COMPLICATIONS

- infection
- malposition
- non-union
- limb shortening
- midfoot or subtalar DJD (contraindication to surgery; potential late complications of surgery)

BELOW-KNEE AMPUTATION

CPT code **27880 amputation, leg, through tibia and fibula**

ICD-9 codes
250.7 diabetes with peripheral circulatory disorders
730.16 chronic osteomyelitis involving lower leg
755.32 longitudinal deficiency of lower limb, NEC; phocomelia
785 symptoms involving cardiovascular system
785.4 gangrene

INDICATIONS

- malignant tumors
- infection
- vascular compromise
- severe open fractures
- congenital malformation (e.g., fibular hemimelia)

ALTERNATIVE TREATMENT

- limb salvage surgery

SURGICAL ANATOMY

Incision

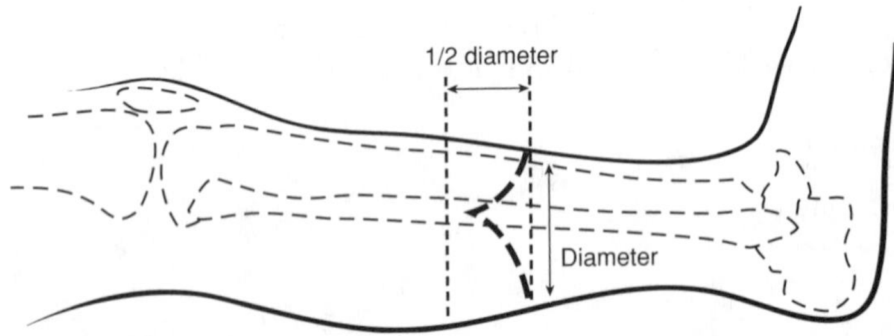

Surgical Techniques

- ideal level is the musculotendinous junction of the gastrocnemius
- ideal bone length is 15 cm distal to the medial tibial articular surface
- supine
- tourniquet
- measure desired length of bone
- outline equal anterior and posterior skin flaps; the length of each flap should equal half the anteroposterior diameter of the leg at the level of the bone cut

- ligate vessels
- divide sharply nerves high to allow retraction away from stump
- bevel anterior tibial cut
- cut fibula 1 cm proximal to the level of the tibial resection
- approximate gastrocnemius–soleus complex to anterior fascia
- drain
- compressive dressing

POSTOPERATIVE MANAGEMENT

- begin stump shrinkage with elastic compressive wrap on postoperative day 2
- begin weight-bearing in temporary prosthesis when wound is healed

REHABILITATION

- prosthetist consultation on postoperative days 1–3
- physical therapy consultation on postoperative day 2 to begin shrink wrapping
- gait training in prosthesis when fitted

COMPLICATIONS

- phantom limb pain
- wound healing
- infection
- poor prosthetic fit due to inadequate tibial length

NOTES

SYME AMPUTATION

CPT code	**27888**	**amputation, ankle, through malleoli of tibia and fibula (e.g., Syme and Pirogoff type procedures), with plastic closures and resection of nerves**
ICD-9 code(s)	**250.7**	**diabetes with peripheral circulatory disorders**
	730.16	**chronic osteomyelitis involving lower leg**
	755.32	**longitudinal deficiency of lower limb, NEC; phocomelia**
	785	**symptoms involving cardiovascular system**
	785.4	**gangrene**

INDICATIONS

- malignant tumors
- infection
- vascular compromise
- severe open fractures
- congenital malformation

ALTERNATIVE TREATMENT

- limb salvage surgery

SURGICAL ANATOMY

Incision

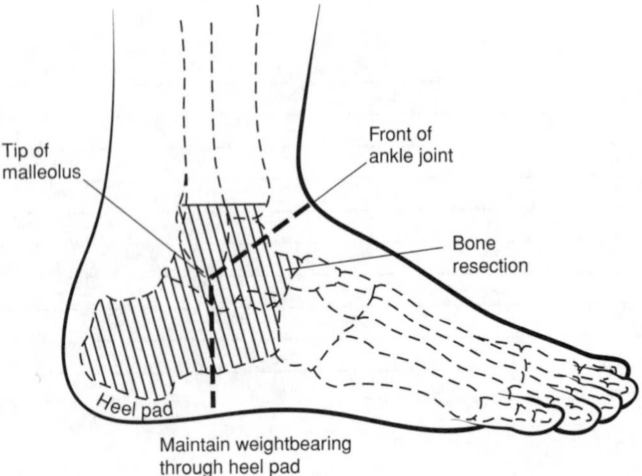

Surgical Techniques

- supine
- tourniquet
- incision to bone
- divide anterior capsule of ankle joint, deltoid ligament, calcaneofibular ligament, posterior ankle joint capsule, and then Achilles tendon
- subperiosteal dissection of the calcaneus
- divide tibia and fibula 0.5 cm proximal to ankle
- dissect medial and lateral plantar nerves and sharply section proximally to cut ends of bone
- section and allow retraction of tendons
- suture deep fascia of heel flap to drill holes in anterior edge of cut tibial surface
- drain
- compressive dressing

POSTOPERATIVE MANAGEMENT

- begin stump shrinkage with elastic compressive wrap on postoperative day 2
- begin weight-bearing in prosthesis when wound is healed

REHABILITATION

- prosthetist consultation on postoperative days 1–3
- gait training in prosthesis when fitted

COMPLICATIONS

- phantom limb pain
- wound healing
- posterior migration of heel pad if not anchored to tibia
- infection

NOTES

TARSAL TUNNEL RELEASE

CPT code **28035 release, tarsal tunnel (posterior tibial nerve decompression)**

ICD-9 code **355.5 tarsal tunnel syndrome**

INDICATIONS

- positive clinical findings with characteristic numbness along the medial and lateral plantar nerve distributions
- failure of conservative care
- positive nerve conduction studies

ALTERNATIVE TREATMENTS

- full-length orthotics, physical therapy, nonsteroidal anti-inflammatory drugs
- look for cause of tarsal tunnel syndrome (e.g., space-occupying lesion) and correct cause
- *beware*: do not release the tarsal tunnel in the face of a pes planus; in that scenario, releasing the tarsal tunnel can significantly worsen symptoms

SURGICAL ANATOMY

- review "classic" nerve distribution of posterior tibial nerve into medial and lateral plantar and calcaneal branches; in reality, often one will find more branches than the classic three because the calcaneal nerve may split into several branches
- "Tom" (tibialis posterior), "Dick" (flexor digitorum longus) and "Harry" (flexor hallucis longus)

Incision

- medial hindfoot: begins 10 cm proximal to tip of medial malleolus, is carried distally parallel to the tibia, and then curves distal and plantar to end at level of the talonavicular joint over the abductor hallucis muscle

APPROACHES

Surgical Techniques

- must carefully release flexor retinaculum
- identify posterior tibial nerve proximally and then trace each nerve off of the main trunk
- medial plantar nerve will pass beneath the abductor hallucis muscle and the lateral plantar nerve will pass behind it
- watch for multiple branches of the calcaneal nerve

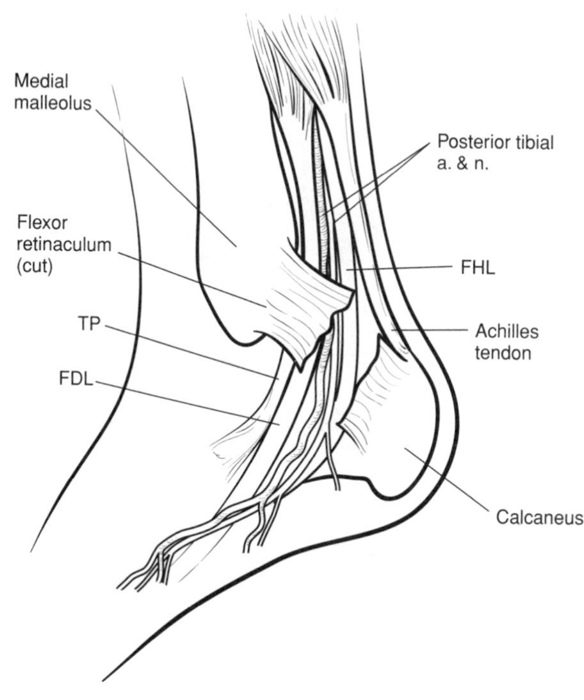

POSTOPERATIVE MANAGEMENT

- keep immobilized for 2–3 weeks, non–weight-bearing on crutches and then WBAT, and begin range of motion exercises

SELECTED REFERENCE

Mann RA, Coughlin MJ. Surgery of the foot and ankle, vol 1, 6th ed. St Louis: CV Mosby, 1986.

NOTES

P A R T   I X

FOOT

PLANTAR FASCIOTOMY

CPT code **28060 fasciectomy, plantar fascia; partial (separate procedure)**

ICD-9 code **728.71 plantar fascitis**

INDICATION

- failure of conservative care for 12 months

ALTERNATIVE TREATMENT

- Achilles tendon stretching program, heel cups, full-length orthotics, nonsteroidal anti-inflammatory drugs, corticosteroid injection, night splints

SURGICAL ANATOMY

- review the structures commonly associated with heel pain: long plantar ligament, plantar fascia, medial plantar nerve, lateral plantar nerve, nerve to the ADQ, and medial calcaneal nerve

Incision

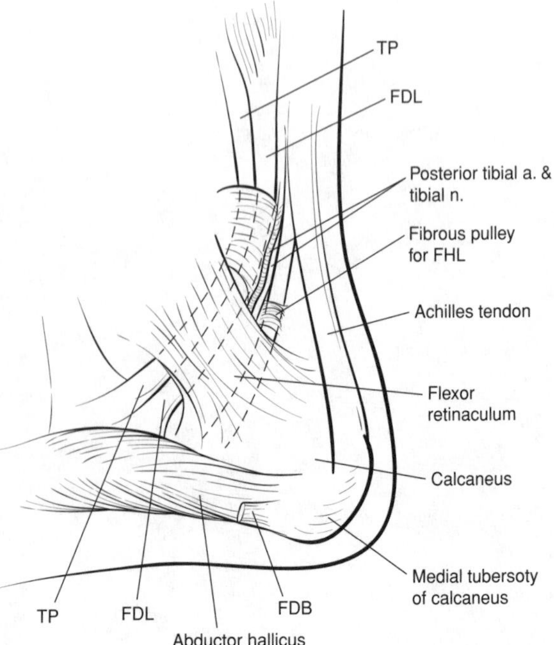

- along the medial side of the heel, curving into the arch just distal to the weight-bearing area of the heel
- care is taken not to injure the medial calcaneal nerve

APPROACHES

Surgical Techniques

- minimal surgical release involves releasing the central slip of the plantar fascia, partial release of the origin of the flexor digitorum brevis (FDB) with or without the calcaneal spur, fascia of the abductor hallucis and quadratus plantae, and the nerve to the ADQ
- in a more aggressive release, the entire posterior tibial nerve is explored with release of all of its branches
- consider tendoachilles lengthening if heel cord is tight

POSTOPERATIVE MANAGEMENT

- SLC non–weight-bearing for 2–4 weeks, followed by weight-bearing in an SLC for 2 weeks
- full activity at 12 weeks

SELECTED REFERENCE

Mann RA, Coughlin MJ. Surgery of the foot and ankle, vol 2, 6th ed. St Louis: CV Mosby, 1996.

NOTES

EXCISION OF MORTON'S NEUROMA

CPT code **28080 excision, interdigital (Morton); neuroma, single, each**

ICD-9 codes **355.6 Morton's neuroma**
355.8 neuropathy leg NEC

INDICATION

- failure of conservative therapy including nonsteroidal anti-inflammatory drugs, Hapad, wide shoes, and interdigital injections

ALTERNATIVE TREATMENTS

- intermetatarsal ligament release
  - 50% long-term success

SURGICAL ANATOMY

- more common between 2nd and 3rd toes than between 3rd and 4th (shown)

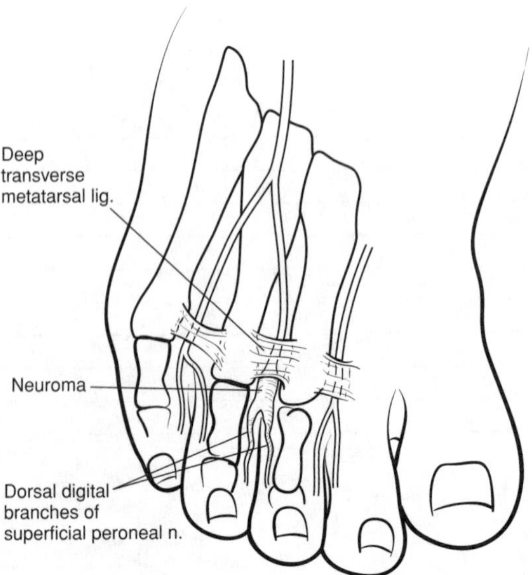

Incision

- 3-cm dorsal web space

APPROACHES

Surgical Techniques

- dissect down to intermetatarsal ligament
- release ligament entirely
- dissect interdigital nerve and branches
- use smooth laminar spreader to visualize
- use plantar pressure to elevate nerve
- release nerve distally
- release plantar branches
- excise nerve proximal to ligament
- closure

POSTOPERATIVE MANAGEMENT

- open toe hard sole shoe for 10 days
- elevate foot for 72 hours

REHABILITATION

- WBAT in hard sole shoe for 10 days
- wean into wider shoe for 2 weeks
- massage scar with vitamin E at 2 weeks

COMPLICATIONS

- infection <1%
- recurrence 5–25%, treated with plantar excision

SELECTED REFERENCES

Haddad S. Compressive neuropathies of the foot and ankle. In: Myerson MS, ed. Foot and ankle disorders. Philadelphia: Saunders, 2002:825–830.

Mann RA, Reynolds JC. Interdigital neuroma; a critical analysis. Foot Ankle Int 1983;3:238–243.

NOTES

EXCISION OF ACCESSORY NAVICULAR BONE

CPT code **28238 reconstruction (advancement), posterior tibial tendon with excision of accessory navicular bone (e.g., Kidner type procedure)**

ICD-9 code **755.67 other anomalies of foot**

INDICATIONS

- 3 types of accessory navicular have been described
  - type I: small accessory bone in the PTT
  - type II: synchondrosis
  - type III: united by a bony bridge
- an accessory navicular is most often symptomatic in adolescence
- indications for surgery include a symptomatic accessory navicular (usually type II) that has failed nonoperative management (orthosis, cast immobilization, or physical therapy)
- consider a bone scan to confirm the diagnosis

ALTERNATIVE TREATMENT

- simple excision of accessory navicular without advancement of tendon

SURGICAL ANATOMY

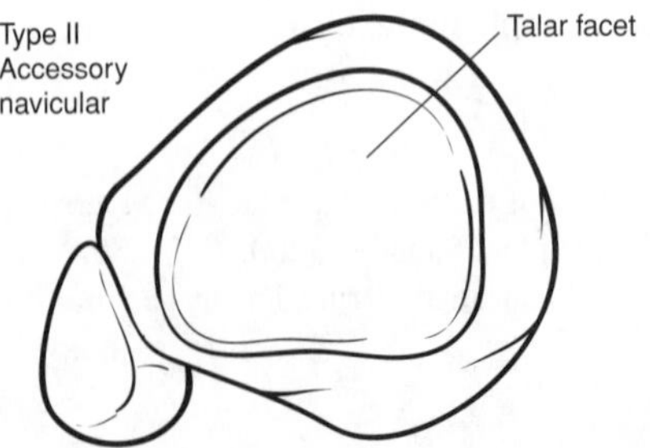

Posterior (proximal) view

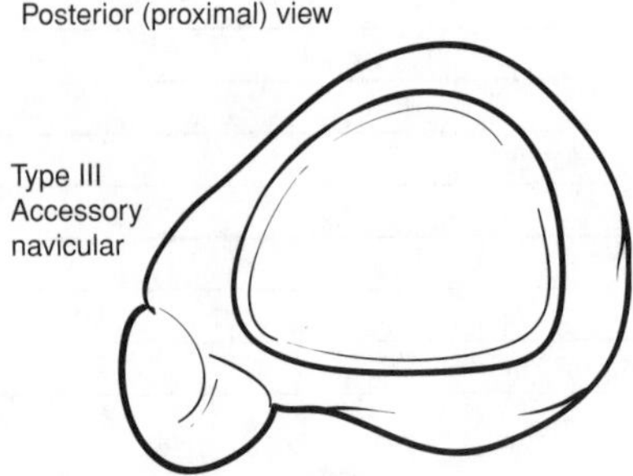

Incision

- longitudinal incision parallel to tibialis posterior (medial malleolus to medial cuneiform)

APPROACHES

Surgical Techniques

- expose posterior tibial tendon insertion
- shell accessory navicular from PTT
- detach PTT insertion from navicular
- resect medial prominence of navicular (flush with medial cuneiform)
- shift tendon plantarly and laterally
- suture tendon to cancellous surface of navicular, or drill hole in navicular and pass the PTT from plantar to dorsal and suture dorsally
- closure

POSTOPERATIVE MANAGEMENT

- SLC with foot inverted, equinus

REHABILITATION

- non–weight-bearing for 3–4 weeks in SLC and then partial weight-bearing for 3–4 weeks in SLC
- full weight bearing at 6–8 weeks
- Kidner's procedure does not necessarily alter the medial longitudinal arch

COMPLICATIONS

- infection
- nerve injury

SELECTED REFERENCES

Coughlin MJ. Sesamoids and accessory bones of the foot. In: Coughlin MJ, Mann RA, eds. Surgery of the foot and ankle. St Louis: CV Mosby, 1999:482–486.

Grogan DP, SI Gasser, Ogden JA. The painful accessory navicular: a clinical and histopathological study. Foot Ankle Int 1989;10:164–169.

NOTES

CORRECTION OF HAMMER TOE OR CLAW TOE

CPT code **28270 metatarsal phalangeal joint release, with or without extensor tenorrhaphy**

ICD-9 codes **735.4 hammer toe acquired**
735.5 claw toe

INDICATIONS

- persistent pain or deformity after conservative treatment with Hapads, wide toe box shoes, orthotics, injections, or nonsteroidal anti-inflammatory drugs
- deformity must be supple

ALTERNATIVE TREATMENTS

- can add PIP arthroplasty (per illustration) (CPT 28285) for rigid contracture
- can add Girdlestone-Taylor tendon transfer (CPT 28285) for instability

SURGICAL ANATOMY

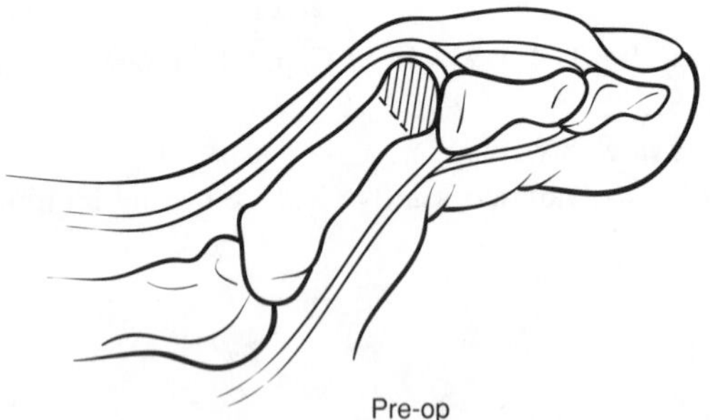

Pre-op

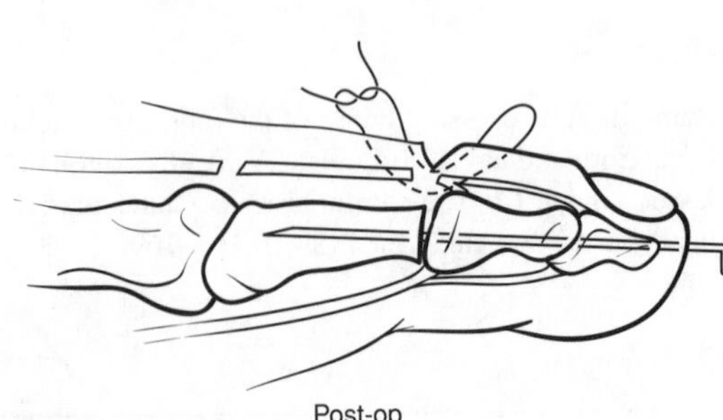

Post-op

Incision

- 3–4-cm dorsal forefoot
- over metatarsal for 1 toe
- over web space for 2 toes

APPROACHES

Surgical Techniques

- dorsal forefoot incision over metatarsal or web space
- isolate EDB tendon and tenotomize with scissors
- isolate EDL tendon and Z-lengthen with knife
- sharply release dorsal MTP capsule
- subperiosteally release collateral ligaments
- release plantar plate
- relocate MTP joint and assess stability
- 0.054-in. K-wires across DIP, PIP, and MTP joints
- repair lengthened EDL
- wound closure

POSTOPERATIVE MANAGEMENT

- heel weight-bearing in hard sole shoe until pin removal
- elevate foot for 72 hours
- remove pin at 4 weeks

REHABILITATION

- full weight-bearing after pin removal
- passive stretching after pin removal
- wide, high toe box shoes

COMPLICATIONS

- infection <1%
- neurovascular compromise 1%
- recurrence 10–50%

SELECTED REFERENCES

Coughlin M, Mann R. Lesser toe deformities. In: Coughlin M., Mann R, eds. Surgery of the foot and ankle, 6th ed. St Louis: Mosby Yearbook, 1993:341–465.

Myerson M, Sheroff M. The pathological anatomy of claw and hammer toes. J Bone Joint Surg 1989;79A:45–49.

NOTES

CORRECTION OF HAMMER TOE

CPT code **28285 correction, hammer toe (e.g., interphalangeal fusion, partial or total phalangectomy)**

ICD-9 codes **735.4 hammer toe acquired (flexion deformity of PIP**
735.5 claw toe acquired (flexion deformity of PIP, extension deformity of MTP)

INDICATIONS

- toe pain and difficulty with shoewear
- not responsive to standard conservative care (shoes with high toe box or soft uppers, doughnut cushions, Budin splint or taping)

ALTERNATIVE TREATMENT

- flexor to extensor tendon transfer (for a flexible hammer toe)

SURGICAL ANATOMY (SEE FIGURE CPT 28270, p. 254.)

Incision

- elliptical incision over PIP joint
- possible longitudinal incision over MTP joint (for extension deformity of MTP joint)

APPROACHES

Surgical Techniques

- elliptical incision over PIP is full thickness (skin, tendon, capsule)
- release collateral ligaments and plantar plate
- resect proximal phalanx head at metaphyseal–diaphyseal junction
- k-wire placement
- address extension contracture at MTP joint if necessary (EDL lengthening, EDB tenotomy, dorsal capsulotomy, MTP arthroplasty)
- closure (includes capsule, extensor tendon, and skin in 1 suture)

POSTOPERATIVE MANAGEMENT

- pin removal at 3 weeks and then tape or splint for 3 weeks

REHABILITATION

- weight-bearing as tolerated
- hard soled shoe
- swelling of toe persists for 1–6 months

COMPLICATIONS

- toe angulation
- recurrence of deformity
- flail toe (too much bone resected)
- infection
- vascular impairment (remove the k-wire)

SELECTED REFERENCES

Coughlin MJ, Dorris J, Polk E. Operative repair of the fixed hammertoe deformity. Foot Ankle Int 2000;21:94–104.

Coughlin M, Mann RA. Lesser toe deformities. In: Coughlin MJ, Mann RA, eds. Surgery of the foot and ankle. St Louis: CV Mosby, 1999:320–391.

NOTES

P A R T X

CASTS & SPLINTS

CLOSED TREATMENT OF CLAVICLE FRACTURE

CPT code **29049 application; figure-of-eight**

ICD-9 code **810.02 closed fracture of shaft of clavicle**

INDICATION

- for comfort with mid 2/3's fracture

ALTERNATIVE TREATMENTS

- prefabricated soft figure-of-eight
- sling

MANAGEMENT

- use for 2–4 weeks for comfort
- begin Codman pendulum exercises in 2–3 weeks

COMPLICATIONS

- pressure sore if applied too tightly
- warn patient about cosmetic "bump" secondary to callus or fracture overlap

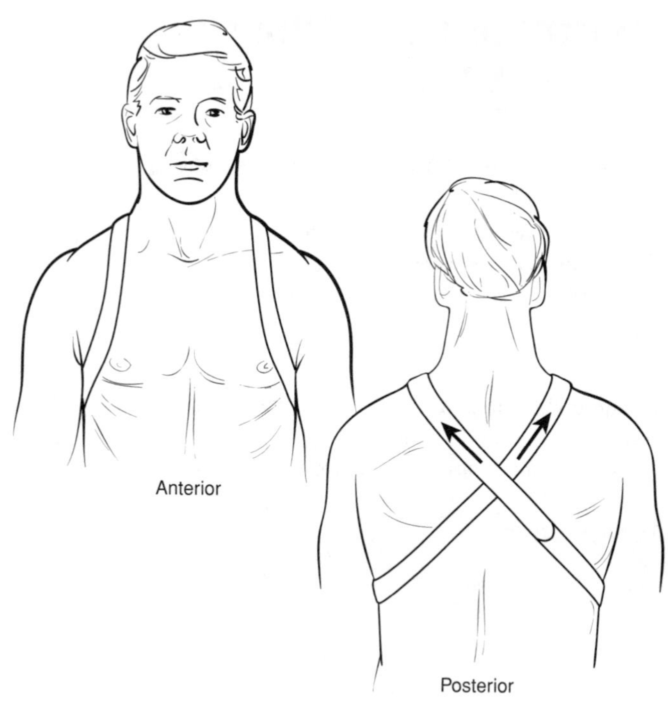

NOTES

APPLICATION OF LONG ARM SUGAR-TONG SPLINT

CPT code **29105 application of long arm splint (shoulder to hand)**

ICD-9 codes
733.11 pathologic fracture of humerus
812.21 shaft of humerus
812.41 supracondylar fracture of humerus

INDICATIONS

- fractures and dislocations of the distal humerus, elbow joint, and proximal forearm requiring immobilization
- postoperative immobilization of the upper extremity

ALTERNATIVE TREATMENTS

- prefabricated long arm splint
- sling

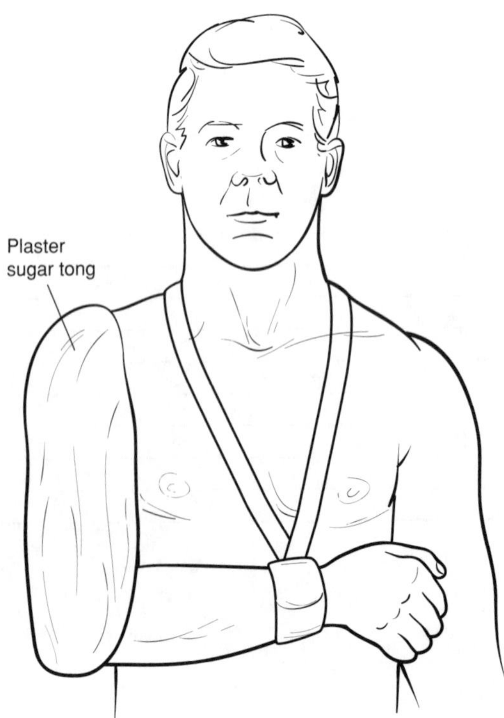

MANAGEMENT

- wrap in compression—as with fracture brace
- x-ray after 2–3 days
- if supracondylar fracture, need to control forearm rotation

COMPLICATIONS

- malunion
- nonunion
- cubitus varus or valgus
- axillary skin maceration

NOTES

APPLICATION OF LONG LEG CAST

CPT code **29345 application of long leg cast (thigh to toes)**

ICD-9 codes **823.20 closed fracture of shaft of tibia**
824 fracture of ankle
821.23 supracondylar fracture of femur

INDICATIONS

- injuries of the lower extremity requiring immobilization including rotational control
- includes bimalleolar fractures of the ankle, tibial and fibular fractures, and injuries of the knee joint

ALTERNATIVE TREATMENTS

- external fixation
- internal fixation
- prefabricated device

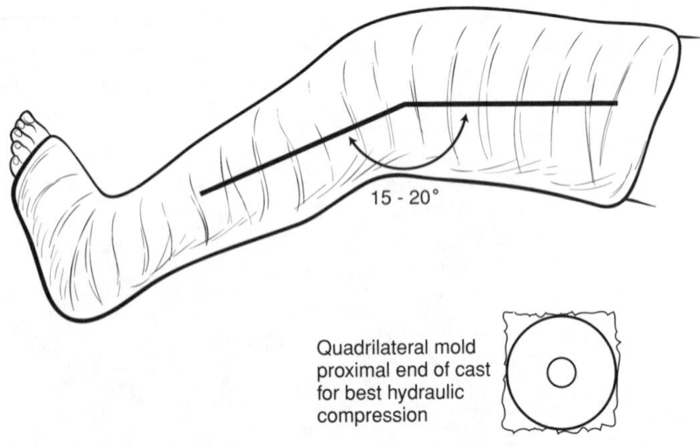

MANAGEMENT

- ensure ankle not in equinus
- extend cast to *groin* for injury at or above knee
- pad heel and peroneal nerve at proximal/lateral fibula

COMPLICATIONS

- skin breakdown
- infection
- neurologic injury
- vascular injury
- DVT
- loss of control of fracture

NOTES

APPLICATION OF CYLINDER CAST

CPT code	**29365**	**application of cylinder cast (thigh to ankle)**
ICD-9 code(s)	**822**	**fracture of patella**
	836.3	**dislocation of patella, closed**
	732.4	**juvenile osteochondrosis of lower extremity (Osgood-Schlatter; Sinding-Larson-Johannson syndrome)**

INDICATION

- injuries or surgical procedures of the knee joint requiring rigid immobilization, where the ankle and foot may remain mobile

ALTERNATIVE TREATMENTS

- well-applied knee immobilizer
- long leg brace
- knee brace

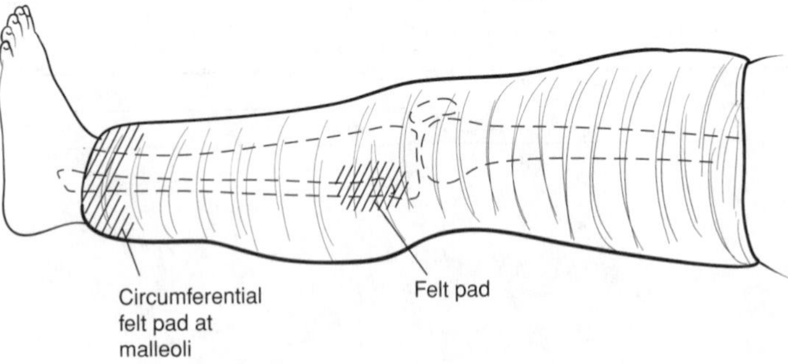

MANAGEMENT

- pad malleoli and proximal fibula
- quadrilateral mold of thigh
- in-shoe stirrup to prevent sliding in patient with “conical” thigh

COMPLICATIONS

- stiffness of the joint
- thromboemboli
- peroneal nerve injury
- irritation or abrasion of ankle soft tissue or pressure sore

NOTES

APPLICATION OF PATELLAR-TENDON BEARING CAST

CPT code **29435 application of patellar tendon bearing cast**

ICD-9 codes **823.20 closed fracture of shaft of tibia**
824 fracture of ankle

INDICATION

- fractures of the tibial shaft requiring immobilization while permitting early weight-bearing

ALTERNATIVE TREATMENTS

- long leg cast
- prefabricated patellar tendon bearing cast

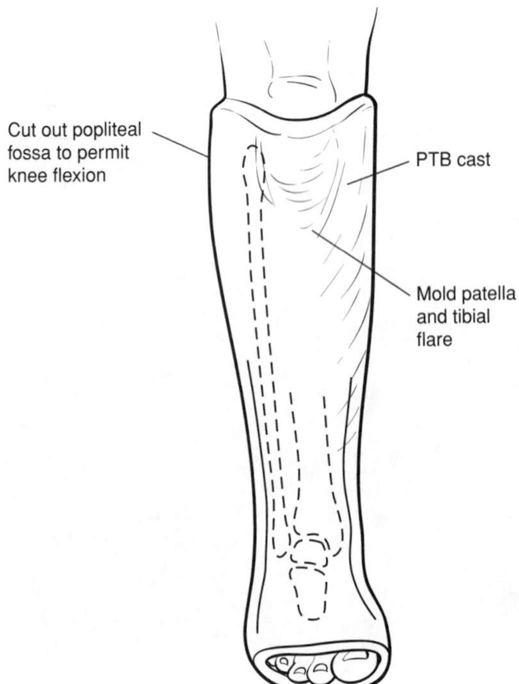

MANAGEMENT

- mold patella and tibial flare to control rotation
- cut out popliteal fossa to permit flexion >90°

COMPLICATIONS

- thromboembolism
- nerve injury
- pressure sores
- delayed union
- non-union

SELECTED REFERENCE

Sarmiento A. A functional below-the-knee cast for tibial fractures. J Bone Joint Surg 1967;49A:855.

NOTES

WEDGING OF CASTS FOR ALIGNMENT

CPT code **29740 wedging of casts (except clubfoot casts)**

INDICATION

- correction of residual angulation after reduction of long bone and application of cast

ALTERNATIVE TREATMENTS

- apply new cast
- use floroscopic x-ray during reduction and application

CONTRAINDICATION

- correction of shortening or displacement

TECHNIQUES

- calculate the wedge on the x-ray, as described by Husted
- hold open wedge with cast padding, cardboard or tongue depressor
- apply layer of plaster or fiberglass
- take another x-ray

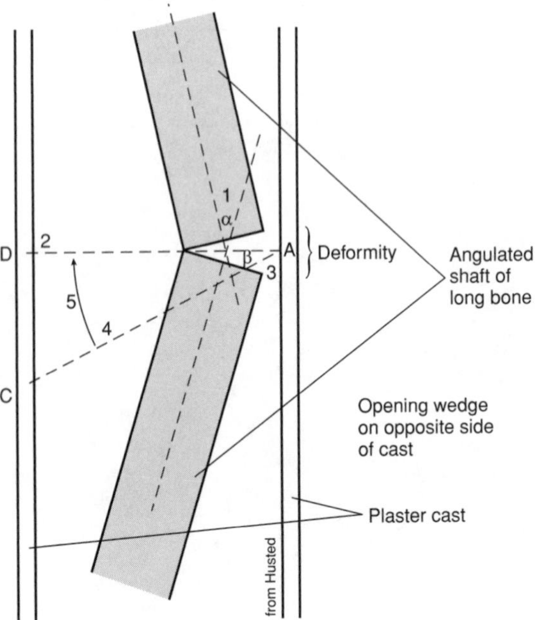

COMPLICATION

- Pressure areas: if large correction is necessary, change the cast

SELECTED REFERENCES

Husted CM. Technique of cast wedging in long bone fractures. Orthop Rev 1986;15:373–378.

Rockwood CA, Green DP, Bucholz RW, Heckman J. Fractures in adults, 4th ed. Philadelphia: Lippincott, 1996.

NOTES

P A R T XI

ARTHROSCOPY

SHOULDER ARTHROSCOPY

CPT code **29815 arthroscopy, shoulder, diagnostic, with or without synovial biopsy (separate procedure)**

ICD-9 codes
718.91 derangement, shoulder
719.41 arthralgia, shoulder
719.21 shoulder synovitis
718.81 instability, shoulder

INDICATIONS

- failure of conservative treatment including nonsteroidal anti-inflammatory drugs, activity modification, and physical therapy
- inconclusive diagnostic testing (rarely)
- evaluation and confirmation of shoulder pathology before open procedures

ALTERNATIVE TREATMENT

- shoulder arthrotomy

SURGICAL ANATOMY

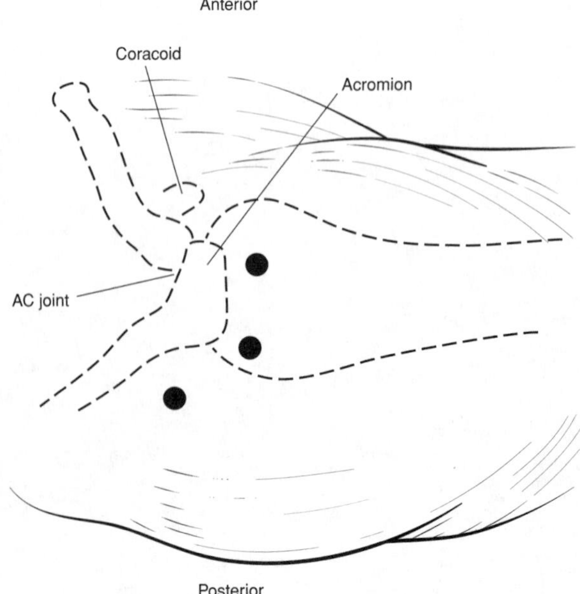

Incision

- portals
  - posterior: 2–3 cm inferior and 1–2 cm medial to posterolateral corner of acromion; standard viewing portal
  - anterior: lateral and superior to coracoid process
  - subacromial: 3 cm distal (lateral) to anterolateral border of the acromion

APPROACHES

- lateral decubitus: 10–15 lbs. of arm traction, with shoulder abduction at 45–60° and forward flexion at 15°
- beach chair and manual traction

Surgical Techniques

- patient positioning
- establish posterior portal
- identify biceps tendon
- establish anterior portal
- probe through anterior portal

POSTOPERATIVE MANAGEMENT

- sling for 1–3 days

REHABILITATION

- depends on operative arthroscopic or open procedure
- if diagnostic only, use sling for 1–3 days and early pendulum exercises; advance to full range of motion and progressive resistive exercises within 1–2 weeks

COMPLICATIONS

- infection
- neurologic injury <0.1%
- chondral damage
- fluid extravasation

SELECTED REFERENCES

Paulos L, Tibone JE, eds. Operative techniques in shoulder surgery. Baltimore: Aspen, 1991.

Weber SC, Abrams JS, Nottage WM. Complications associated with arthroscopic shoulder surgery. Arthroscopy 2002;18:88–95.

KNEE ARTHROSCOPY

CPT code	**29870**	**arthroscopy, knee, diagnostic, with or without synovial biopsy (separate procedure) (usually therapeutic)**
ICD-9 codes	**717.9**	**internal derangement, unspecified, knee**
	719.16	**hemoarthrosis, knee**
	719.26	**knee synovitis**

INDICATIONS

- evaluation and confirmation before knee arthrotomy
- evaluation for chronic knee synovitis
- second-look procedure to assess healing for meniscal repair or cartilage transplantation procedures
- contraindication to other diagnostic procedure, i.e., magnetic resonance imaging

ALTERNATIVE TREATMENTS

- diagnostic radiology: magnetic resonance imaging or arthrography
- arthrotomy

SURGICAL ANATOMY

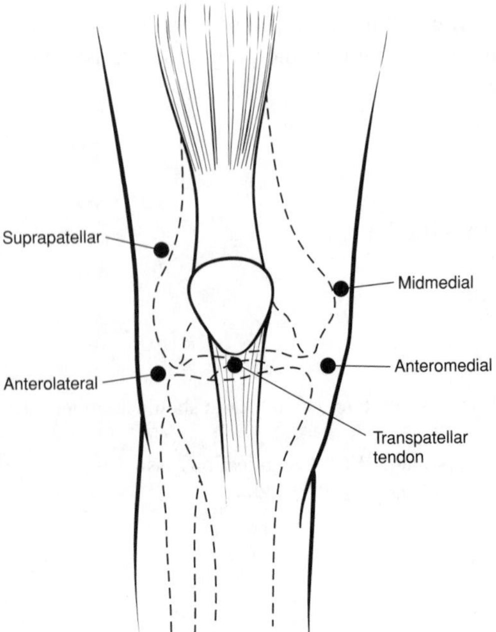

Incision

standard portals

- anteromedial
- suprapatellar
- anterolateral
- midmedial

APPROACHES

- supine positioning: leg holder with both knees flexed or lateral swivel post with the operated leg off to the side

Surgical Techniques

- establish portals
- insertion of 30° arthroscope
- connect inflow via gravity flow or pump
- attach fiberoptic light source
- establish outflow
- inspect and probe

POSTOPERATIVE MANAGEMENT

- compressive bandage
- crutches for 2–3 days

REHABILITATION

- ankle pumps
- straight leg raises
- quadriceps sets
- weight-bearing as tolerated

COMPLICATIONS

- overall <2%
- instrument breakage
- hemarthrosis 1%
- thromboembolism
- infection <0.25%
- neurologic injury <0.1%
- iatrogenic chondral damage
- vascular injury
- synovial fistula

SELECTED REFERENCES

Delis KT, Hunt N, Strachan RK, Nicolaides AN. Incidence, natural history and risk factors of deep vein thrombosis in elective knee arthroscopy. Thromb Haemost 2001;86:817–821.

Orthopaedic Grand Grouonds on CD-ROM, Series II—Arthroscopy. American Academy of Orthopaedic Surgery, Rosemont, 1998.

Wind WM, McGrath BE, Mindell ER. Infection following knee arthroscopy. Arthroscopy 2001:17:878–883.

NOTES

PART XII

LUMBAR PUNCTURE

LUMBAR PUNCTURE

CPT code	**62270 spinal puncture, lumbar, diagnostic**
ICD-9 codes	**324.1 intraspinal abscess**
	320 bacterial meningitis

INDICATIONS

- suspected meningitis
- other diagnostic problems, e.g., suspected central nervous system infection or neoplasm

SURGICAL ANATOMY

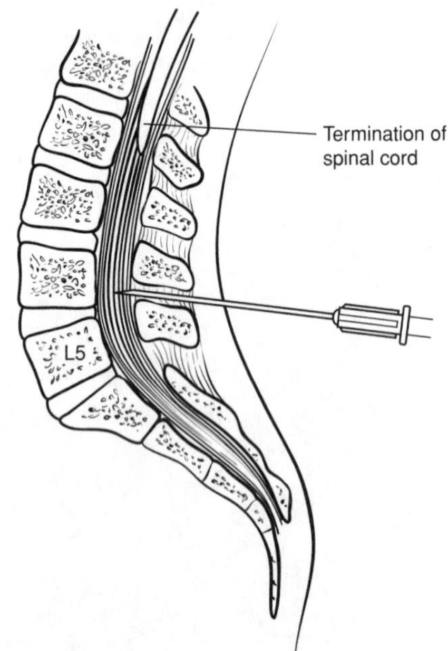

APPROACHES

Surgical Techniques

- patient in decubitus position
- hips, knees, and neck flexed and held by assistant
- in children, presedation is essential
- angle spinal needle at approximately 30° cephalad between spinous processes

- free flow of cerebrospinal fluid is expected; bloody aspirate suggests epidural venous bleed
- volume of cerebrospinal fluid should be based on patient size and diagnostic requirements: e.g., adult versus child

POSTOPERATIVE MANAGEMENT

- postpuncture headaches are rare; limit activity for 1–2 hours after aspiration

COMPLICATIONS

- headache occurs in <5%
- persistent headache, i.e., >2 days, may require blood patch by anesthesiologist

NOTES

INDEX

G

H